Safe and Sound

Healthy Travel with Children

Marlene M. Coleman, M.D.

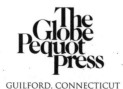
The
Globe
Pequot
Press

GUILFORD, CONNECTICUT

To Bill with love.
For your sense of humor . . .
for past and future
healthful travel together.

Text design: Linda Loiewski

Library of Congress Cataloging-in-Publication Data

Coleman, Marlene.
   Safe and sound : healthy travel with children / Marlene M. Coleman.
     p. cm.
   Includes index.
   ISBN 0-7627-2691-1
     1. Children—Health and hygiene. 2. Travel—Health aspects. I. Title.

RJ47 .C655 2003
613.6'8'083—dc21

                                       2002033913

Manufactured in the United States of America
First Edition/First Printing

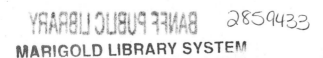

Contents

Acknowledgments

The collaborative effort with gifted people is the real joy in completing a book. Thank you all for making this book possible.

My special thanks with love go to my family—in particular, my dearest mother for always encouraging and believing in me; my twin sister, Darlene, for her love and expertise; my talented and caring children, Charlyn, Matthew, and Damon; I remember with joy the trips I took with my late father, my brothers Denver and Kent, and the rest in my family; and to my husband, Bill, for his unwavering love.

My great appreciation goes to my colleagues at Caltech, USC Medical School, and Harbor Pediatrics; Leslie Kossoff for her friendship and guidance; Laurie Harper for her expertise in the publishing industry; and for their editorial and administrative support, Amy Booth, Pat Hatton, Lou Hoover, Warren Jameson, and Judy Kleinberg.

It is an honor to be associated with The Globe Pequot Press. In particular, Executive Editor Mary Norris shared her vision for my book throughout the process. My thanks go as well to her excellent team, including Paula Brisco and Ellen Urban.

Throughout the book I have tried to express the passion that I have had for more than twenty-five years for taking care of children, adolescents, and college students in travel situations. My great hope is that readers everywhere will share my passion for travel with children and open up their worlds even farther.

Introduction

There is nothing in life more precious than our children. We love and protect them and want to make sure they are healthy and safe at all times. We want them to have rich lives, full of memorable experiences. It is not surprising that we want to share with them the rewards and discoveries of travel.

Now is a great time to travel with your family. The travel industry—airlines, cruise companies, hotels, resorts, tour operators, and a great many destinations—have begun to take family travel seriously. Where once the prime audience was singles or retired people, today the industry recognizes that many families, even those with very young children, are travelers. In fact, when both parents work, a family vacation may be a rare and valuable opportunity to enjoy quality time together.

Traveling with children—or even one child—involves complications adults never face when traveling alone. With proper preparation, however, travel with your children can result in a series of wonderfully rewarding experiences. Healthy travel is not just concerned with disease but also with the psychology of well-being and the prevention of physical injury.

Why Travel with Children?

There are probably as many reasons to travel as there are trips to be taken. We share many of them in common. Here are a few:

- Travel involves the adventure and excitement of meeting new people, exploring new vistas, and savoring new cultures. The repetitive groove of daily life can entangle any of us in its mind-deadening grasp. Travel is stim-ulating and can help dispel any boredom or malaise we might feel.

- Travel can awaken and inspire us to rediscover our true passions. Taking ourselves out of our daily routines gives us the time to examine our priorities and decide what is really important to us.

- Travel reminds us of who gives meaning to our lives. It gives us a fresh outlook and ultimately a renewed appreciation for the important people in our lives.

- Travel helps us dispel misconceptions and prejudices we may have regarding other cultures and people. Travel broadens our worldview and gives us new appreciation for the amazing variety of precious life on the planet that we share with each other.

- Travel expands our personal power by increasing our knowledge of exciting and different cultures. We discover enhanced expression and creativity within ourselves, making us more attractive to others.

- Travel is the surest cure for that "trapped" feeling. A change of context makes our moods and attitudes more positive and exhilarating.

- Travel enhances our sense of independence and confidence. Through it we attain feelings of personal power over our lives.

- Travel gives us new topics of conversation to share with others. Everything we see and learn in our travels stimulates new ideas that make us more interesting and knowledgeable.

- Travel can give us time to be pampered and allow us to relax. In our daily lives it is easy to forget the restorative value of relaxation. If we permit it to work its magic, travel will give us the opportunity to fully relax.

Whatever your reasons for leaving home, travel can bring renewed inspiration and personal enlightenment. It can fuel growth within ourselves and in our relationships with fellow travelers—especially family members. As we relax and become acquainted with new people and places, we can dispel stress and open new pathways to our dreams.

Your travel experience starts long before you leave home. It begins in your imagination, perhaps sparked by a photo, a story in a magazine, or a friend's tales of his or her journey. Some of us may be able to take off on a whim, but most of us have to strategize the needs of work and family before we can leave home.

When our children are part of our travels, we need to take additional steps to ensure their comfort and safety. This book is your guide to those steps, starting with these:

1. Start your planning and preparation as early as possible. Take it as far as you can as soon as you can. This will prevent the exhausting last-minute push to get everything done, which often means some important details get overlooked.

2. Get everything ready the day before departure so that when D-day arrives, you can start your trip rested, relaxed, and ready for fun.

3. Become mentally and physically prepared to protect your family against any hazards you may encounter.

4. Involve the entire family in planning and preparing for an enriching trip, in taking photos and collecting other reminders of your travels, and in reliving those memories at family gatherings.

If you are expecting a child or thinking about having one, or even if you have one or half a dozen already, this book will help you to take the right steps and make the right decisions as you plan to travel together. Read it with highlighter in hand and pen and paper at your side. Take lots of notes and update them after this trip and before the next.

The preparation you do for this trip will help you on every trip you take in the future. Bon voyage!

Part I

Travel Planning, Safety, and Well-being

Chapter 1
Planning a Vacation

As every parent knows, a trip with children (even to the grocery store!) is more complex and demanding than traveling alone. But with wise planning and preparation it can also be far more rewarding. Thorough planning has always been important; for today's travelers with children it is imperative. These pages will suggest many ways to make your family travels healthier, safer, more fun, and less of a hassle.

The world has far more safe, fascinating, and delightful places to visit than anyone has time to enjoy in a lifetime. With a little planning and forethought, you and your children will soon be on your way to discovering them for yourselves.

Ten Basic Health and Safety Suggestions

1. Learn as much as you can about your destination and activities and plan ahead.

2. Prepare for routine conditions and emergencies and do everything possible to avoid hazards.

3. Find out how to access medical help and carry important phone numbers.

4. Assemble a first-aid kit and learn how to use it.

5. Dress comfortably.

6. Drink plenty of water and eat well.

7. Get enough sleep.

8. Pace yourself.

9. Keep your sense of humor and remember that even the best-laid plans can fall apart.

10. Have a great trip!

Preplanning

Before we talk about planning, or even preplanning, let's take a moment to con-sider how you are going to do your travel planning. If you are computer-savvy, you may want to keep your notes on the computer. If so, create a separate folder for "Travel," and within that, a folder for this trip by destination or date. Every time you add something to your information, make sure it goes into your trip folder. Keep your notes in separate files by subject (for example, "Lists," "Camping," "Transportation," "Medical," "Paris," "Yellowstone," and so forth).

If the computer is not an option—and even if it is—you should have a notebook or file for papers. You will accumulate brochures, maps, articles, correspondence, and lots of notes related to your trip. Accordion files work well, or a large three-ring binder might be a good solution. Your other planning equipment should include a writing pad, pens and pencils, highlighters, and scissors (for cutting out articles).

When you take notes (or clip articles)—on paper or electronically—date your notes and jot down the source of information. That will help to keep your papers in order and will be especially useful if you need additional information—now or later.

You may already know exactly where you are going on your trip—perhaps a visit to grandparents or a weekend in the mountains. More likely, you have lots of ideas about how you would like to fill those few days or weeks you have set aside. Choosing a destination may be one of the biggest challenges you face.

Preplanning helps you gather essential information so you can make good decisions about your trip. So let's get started. Get your pencil and paper (or sit down at the computer) and begin your preplanning list by writing down the follow-ing information about your upcoming trip:

- Who will be going? List everyone, including family, friends, nannies, and pets, as appropriate.

- What are the dates of travel? Include days of the week for your starting and ending dates. What season is it?

- Where are you going (if you know)?

- How will you get there? You may not know the answer to this question yet, but write down your options (for example, drive, fly, or take a train).

- How will you get around once you are there? Will you need to rent a vehicle?

- Where will you stay?

- What kind of activities would you and your family enjoy most? Include as many as you can think of—remember, this is just preplanning—and don't forget hobbies and special interests.

- What limitations do you have to consider in your planning? Think about medical conditions, allergies, physical limitations, fitness, energy levels, ages, weather, time constraints, and any other factors than might influence your decisions.

- What is your travel budget?

As you begin to consider your options, refer to your preplanning list. You may discover that you have left something out or that you were too ambitious when you made your initial list. That's why you plan. Edit your list accordingly. Better to discover the problems early on paper than when you and your family are far from home.

Choosing a Destination

Family travel can and should be packed with enriching experiences and great fun. Ideally your destination will be rewarding for everyone in your party. It will offer a safe and healthy combination of activities and relaxation, group and private time, and enough variety to meet everyone's needs.

If your children live in the city most of the year, taking them to visit family or friends who live in rural places can be an exciting adventure for them. Having lots of space to roam around in can give them many memorable experiences—or expose them to risks they would never encounter at home. Equally, if your children live with you in the country, a visit to the city can involve both adventures and hazards. As you choose a destination, be aware of your children's inexperience in the unfamiliar environment.

Your choice of a destination is influenced by some of the factors you included in your preplanning list: length of time, season, budget, interests, and previous travel experience. Here are some additional considerations:

- Do you want to stay in hotels or motels, camp, or stay with friends or relatives?

- Are you interested in indoor (museums, for example) or outdoor (hiking, theme parks) activities, or both?

- Will you need to be with your child at all times, or will you be able to arrange for child care and some "adult" time on your own?

- If you have not traveled with your child before, are you willing to take a short "test" trip?

With those considerations in mind, make a preliminary list of destinations. Talk to your friends. Look at magazines and on-line information about the places you are considering. Discuss the options with your family. There are many places to find travel information:

- Go to your local library. It may not have the most current information on destinations, but it probably has large-format photography books that might be helpful.

- Examine Web sites that describe the places you plan to visit. (See Appendix C.)

- Obtain current maps of the cities where you will be staying and study them. You can find maps on-line, at the auto club, and at travel stores and bookstores.

- For destinations in the United States, you can request information from the chambers of commerce in the cities you are considering.

- For destinations outside the United States, check with the Centers for Disease Control and Prevention (CDC)—www.cdc.com—and the U.S. Department of State—www.state.gov—for health and travel advisories.

- Go to a quality bookstore and get the most recently published and information-rich books available.

While you are researching destinations, investigate the safety conditions—both disease and disorder—in every area on your itinerary. Also, consider the weather. Look for typical weather patterns, including storm seasons (hurricanes, tornadoes) and temperatures. Researching weather patterns cannot guarantee blue skies and gentle breezes, but it can greatly reduce your risk of spending your vacation storm-bound in a hotel with restless youngsters.

Once you have narrowed down your choices, you may want to talk with a travel agent (see below), but first you should probably evaluate whether your children are ready to take this trip.

Are Your Children Travel-Worthy?

Are your children travel-worthy in the sense that a ship is seaworthy or an airplane is airworthy? If there is doubt in your mind about your children's travel-worthiness, approach lengthy or out-of-country travel with caution.

What makes a child travel-worthy? Being willing to follow your instructions quickly without argument. Being able to control impulsive behavior. Having patience with minor inconveniences. (This, of course, is too much to expect of infants, but toddlers should be able to understand that their wants cannot always be met instantly.)

Many parents inadvertently train their children to ignore what they tell them. They say "Don't" with no intention of enforcing their command or issue a mind-numbing stream of warnings when there's no real danger. Children recognize this and do as they please. If a child constantly hears a parent say, "Be careful" or "Watch out," he or she soon decides the warnings are not worth listening to. This can have disastrous results when the danger is life threatening.

The word "No" should be used only in situations where instant obedience is vital to the child's safety. When you want your child to stop doing something that is merely annoying, use other words such as, "Stop that," "Quit it," and so on.

If you get an appropriate response to your "No," reward the child with a loving hug. If your "No" is not obeyed promptly, punish the child appropriately. Explain the importance of your instructions. Bright, energetic, but unruly children often need to be told why obedience is important for their, or the family's, safety. A grueling interrogation as to precisely why they did not follow instructions often makes a more lasting impression than grounding or spanking does.

Lay down intelligent guidelines and children will follow them, particularly when the family is in unfamiliar territory. Children who live in a warm and encouraging environment generally want to please their parents.

If your children are not travel-worthy, do not expect them to become instantly compliant on a trip. First change your parenting habits, because they are probably the primary source of obedience problems. Tighten discipline by giving children fewer but more meaningful instructions. Then allow them a few weeks to get accustomed to your new regime before leaving home.

It is natural for teenagers to seek independent activities and prize opportunities to make their own decisions. As loving parents, seek to guide rather than blindly oppose their efforts to find their own way. Bear in mind that they are approaching adulthood in today's cultural climate, which may be quite different from the one you experienced as an adolescent. Your task—and it is not an easy one—is to help teenagers avoid the serious calamities of life without stifling their opportunities to live life to the fullest as they, not you, define that goal.

Should You Take a Nanny?

Depending on how many adults will be going, the number and ages of your children, the activities you have planned, and your budget, you might want to consider adding a child care companion to your family trip. That person could be a relative or friend of the family, a nanny, an au pair, or a baby-sitter who already knows your children well.

If you will be traveling alone with your child or children—especially if you will be working during your trip—a baby-sitter you already know can provide both child care and peace of mind. If you and your spouse hope to have some time alone, an extra adult—even a young adult—can give you a break from full-time parenting. If you have physical limitations, a companion can allow your children to participate in more vigorous activities than you would choose.

Although you may be able to find a local sitter through your hotel, you and your children both will likely be more comfortable with someone tried and true. Remember that traveling with someone is one of the toughest tests of compatibility. Do not assume that your mild-mannered baby-sitter or your teenage cousin will be a perfect traveling companion. Testing compatibility on a weekend jaunt could prevent a disaster on your hard-earned vacation.

The physical and financial arrangements also may vary, so make sure everyone understands the details before you leave home. You will be expected to pay for transportation, room, and board, but will you need to pay a salary in addition to expenses? Will your caregiver require a separate room? Grandma might not be so happy to accompany you on your summer vacation if she knows she will be the built-in baby-sitter. On the other hand, a young cousin or neighbor might see full-time baby-sitting for your brood as a very worthwhile exchange for a month in Europe.

If you decide to take along a child care companion, remember that he or she also will need to be diligent regarding health care, vaccinations, packing, and other preplanning concerns. Discuss beforehand time-off arrangements, activities, rules, money, and how you will deal with emergencies. Bringing along a companion for your children can add immeasurably to your vacation enjoyment if you begin your planning well in advance and talk openly about your plans as they take shape.

Involve Your Children in Trip Planning

To get the most benefit from the fun and mind-expanding value of travel, let your children participate in planning the trip. The more you allow your children to help set up the trip, the less complaining and whining you are likely to hear. More importantly, the entire family will enjoy a more relaxing and enriching trip when the children are meaningfully involved along the way.

As you are considering your itinerary, discuss some of the options available at each destination and have your children make a preliminary list of the things they would like to do. When you get there, choose some activities from their list and some from yours. And don't forget that both of your lists will probably change as you discover new possibilities: Who knew that there would be a surfing exhibition or elephant rides?

When your children have had some experience choosing vacation activities, try giving them a budget for a weekend family car trip. Let them pick the destination and lodgings and choose your family's activities. To instill a sense of responsibility and foresightedness, limit your parental vetoes to potential disasters. Allowing children to make mistakes and live with the consequences or to succeed on their own can teach valuable lessons.

Where Will You Stay?

Although family vacations tend to emphasize daytime activities, nighttime comfort is every bit as important. Depending on the number and age of your children, the type of vacation experience you are planning, and your budget, your options generally include camping, visiting the homes of friends or relatives, or staying in motels, hotels, or resorts.

As you evaluate your options, consider and write down your answers to the following questions:

- Will the entire family share a room or will you need two or more adjoining or separate rooms? How many beds and what sizes will you need? Who will share rooms?

- Can everyone in your party share a bathroom? If not, how many baths will you need?

- Does anyone in your party require special equipment, such as wheelchair access, cribs, or bed rails?

- If you are traveling with an infant, will you need diaper service?

- Would you prefer to prepare some or all of your meals yourself, or will you be eating every meal in a restaurant?

- Do your overnight accommodations need to be close to the daytime activities you have planned?

- If you arrive by plane, how will you get from the airport to your overnight destination? (Some hotels offer shuttle services, which may be safer than taxis.)

- How long will you stay in each place? (Count every night you will be away, even if one or more of the nights will be spent on planes or in airports.)

- If you stay with friends, do you have a backup plan in case the arrangements do not work out?

- If you are camping or staying in someone's home, what will you do if one of your companions gets sick?

Creepers and toddlers are curious little people who will get into anything they can reach and put everything they can grab in their mouths. Before making plans to stay with your children as guests in someone else's home, you need to consider three matters:

1. Is the house in question adequately childproofed for the ages of your children?

2. Is your relationship with your hosts strong enough—and are they genial enough—to permit you to check their home for hazards to your children?

3. Will your hosts make, or permit you to make, the changes you believe are essential for your children's safety?

If the answer to any of these questions is "No," consider whether staying at a nearby motel or hotel would put less strain on the relationship and be safer for your little ones.

In selecting hotels, motels, resorts, and even campgrounds, ask your friends, the auto club, and a travel agent for recommendations. Brochures and Web sites may be helpful in providing descriptions, but remember that they are designed to sell the accommodations, not offer an impartial look at the facility. The auto club and reputable guidebooks have rating systems that evaluate accommodations based on a specific set of standards. Once you have narrowed your choices, call and talk to a reservation agent or manager at the facility. The service you get on the phone will probably be a good indication of the kind of service you can expect when you are a guest.

It is always a good idea to have a backup plan in case your original arrangements do not work out as expected. Just knowing the name and phone number of a second motel nearby will give you considerable peace of mind.

Your Family Vacation Ally: The Travel Agent

With all of today's on-line self-booking options, you may be thinking of handling your own reservations. But an experienced and knowledgeable agent can make your trip easier and provide you with valuable information and services.

If you don't already have a travel agent, start by asking your friends who travel with their children for recommendations. Look for an agent who has a track record in the industry and is well traveled, creative, and willing to do whatever it takes to find the best solution to your travel challenge. Once you find promising prospects, visit their offices, if possible, and have a conversation that includes the following:

• Find out how long the person has been in the travel industry and how long he or she has been an agent.

- Does the agent have knowledge about traveling with children? More and more destinations and tour operators offer programs designed for children and families; an agent who is well versed in the most current offerings is a tremendous asset. Hotel and transportation practices and pricing for families vary widely; you should be able to count on your agent for sound advice.

- If you or a family member has physical limitations, a knowledgeable travel agent with experience in special-needs travel is very important.

- Ask whether the agency is a "preferred supplier" for particular cruise companies, tour operators, hotels, or airlines. (If the agent doesn't handle your airline of choice, he or she will have a hard time satisfying your needs.)

- Ask whether the agent has visited your destination (and when) and whether he or she has sent other travelers there (and how many). Will the agent be able to make recommendations on lodgings, attractions, and restaurants?

- If you inquire about the agent's favorite destination worldwide, that might give you more insight into his or her personality.

- Will the agent be booking through a tour operator or directly with airlines and hotels?

As you ask your questions, observe whether the agent is really listening to you and giving you thoughtful answers. Does he or she continually let phone calls interrupt your conversation? The way the agent talks to people on the phone and in the office is the way he or she will talk to you. Is that okay?

Your association with a travel agent is a relationship. You will work together on your travel plans. Any advance preparation you do will make you a more desirable customer and will help you obtain superior service and advice. You need to feel comfortable with and have trust in the travel agent and be willing to share your worries as well as your hopes for your trip. By asking the right questions, you can add a valuable member to your travel team.

Passports, Visas, Customs, Credit, and Other Concerns

If you are going out of the country, you will need a passport. U.S. passports are issued for a ten-year period for adults. If you are applying for your first passport, unexpected problems may develop in proving your eligibility. The Department of State generally issues passports within about six weeks, but to be on the safe side, apply at least ninety days before you plan to go. (If there is an error on your newly issued passport, you may have to reapply.) If you encounter a last-minute emergency, the passport office will expedite your application for an additional fee, but it will still take a minimum of two weeks.

If your child is under the age of fourteen, you must provide additional documentation. See the "Special Requirements" page at the Department of State passport Web site for complete details: travel.state.gov/specialreq.html.

If you have a passport but it will expire before or during your trip, allow plenty of time to get it renewed before you leave. Security considerations have slowed passport processing.

When you travel, take along an extra passport photo and two copies of the first two pages of your passport (with photo, personal information, and signature) and keep them in a safe place, separate from your passport.

Many foreign destinations require visas; apply for these early at the country's embassy in Washington, D.C., or at a nearby consulate. Consulates may keep limited hours and there may be more than one visit required to secure visas, so allow plenty of time before your departure.

If you plan to take foreign-made items (such as a laptop or camera) out of the United States, or if you plan to purchase items in a foreign country, it would be wise to research U.S. Customs duties and exemptions. You can access the U.S. Customs Web site at www.customs.ustreas.gov/travel/travel.htm and order its helpful brochure.

Pack a large manila envelope in your carry-on and put all your purchase receipts in it. If you have to go through customs, you will be happy to have them all in one place. (Those large envelopes are also great for the postcards, maps, and brochures you collect along the way; take a few.)

Credit cards are widely accepted in most major cities throughout the world and are convenient for hotel, transportation, and travel purchases. Check your credit limit on each card you carry and stay within that limit; exceeding the limit on an international purchase can turn a simple transaction into a complicated tangle. On your list of important phone numbers, carry the toll-free lost-card number for your credit card service.

Clothing Comfort and Style

In earlier centuries, fashion ignored comfort and convenience. If acres of petticoats, restrictive jackets, or pinching shoes were fashionable at home, they would be equally fashionable on the road. Today it is not stylish to be uncomfortable.

Inexperienced travelers tend to overpack and typically wear only a few of the outfits they have brought along. Visualize every situation you and your children will be in and decide what clothing you will need.

Remember that you will be with other travelers who have the same luggage limitations, so you do not need to bring a vast wardrobe. Less is better than more, especially when you are rushing to catch a plane. Think twice about two garments that serve the same purpose, and leave one of them at home.

Packing Tips

- Select trip clothing that you and your children will be comfortable in.

- Check with a travel agent, consulate, or visitors bureau to find out whether there are any restrictions or expectations regarding proper attire. (For instance, if you plan to visit a tribal village in Fiji, shorts and halter tops are not appropriate. In many parts of the world, a man in shorts is not considered fully dressed.)

- Choose lightweight garments that can be worn (or removed) in layers and will be appropriate for more than one occasion.

- Select shoes that will be comfortable for walking longer distances than you and your children may walk at home.

- Break in shoes thoroughly before you go.

- Clothing should be wash-and-wear for easy maintenance. Test-wash clothing before you leave home to be sure wrinkles and shrinkage are not a problem. Although cotton clothing may be the most comfortable in hot, humid conditions, even small garments may take more than twenty-four hours to air-dry if you do not have access to a clothes dryer.

Photography, Souvenirs, and Shopping

One of the great pleasures of travel is bringing home memories and gifts. With a little planning, and a little attention as you go, you will not only create long-lasting memories, but you will also help your children become more observant, informed, and enthusiastic travelers. Here are some thoughts on successful memory-making. Try a few of these ideas and add your own. Some will be more suitable if you are driving, others will work on almost any trip. Vary your activities from day to day. And have fun!

- Bring cameras for everyone—but not for every day. Your family may have a designated photographer, but why not let everyone in on the fun? With easy-to-use disposable cameras readily available, you can turn anyone into "photographer for a day." (Remember that it is courteous to ask permission before taking someone's picture. And with increased concerns about security, photos may be prohibited at some locations, such as military/government buildings, bridges, and airports.)

- Take along a small tape recorder and let the kids interview each other and people you meet on your trip. In addition to talking about your adventures, you can also create group stories: Someone starts the story and then each person adds a sentence or two before handing the recorder to the next person. (This is a great—and usually quite amusing—way to pass the time on long driving trips.)

- Try your hand at something colorful. Pack some crayons, watercolors, pens, or pastels along with some small sketch pads. Instead of always using the camera, try sketching. Make sure to date and identify the drawings. Give each child his or her own sketch pad and be sure that you participate, too. (Parents who protest that they "can't draw" will soon have children imitating their reluctance. Parents who draw enthusiastically, even if with little skill, allow their children to discover their own creativity without fear. And remember—everyone's skills improve with practice!) Be generous with your praise.

- Pack a few "favors" in your suitcase. Select items that are not too heavy to carry. A little surprise gift now and then makes everyone feel great. It could be a food treat, a trinket, a T-shirt, a puzzle, a bookmark, or a tiny treasure from your last stop.

- Give each person a blank book such as an inexpensive, unlined composition book, and have him or her create a trip log, complete with sketches, notes, diary entries, and souvenirs collected along the way. (A small pair of scissors, glue stick, and tape will make this project easier.)

- Bring postage stamps and mailing labels that you've pre-addressed to your children's friends. Encourage your kids to select, write, and send postcards.

- Share a book. See if you can find a book that relates to your destination and spend part of each day or evening reading it aloud to the whole family.

- Buy someone a gift. Before you set out, make a list of gifts you would like to bring home—and don't forget early birthday and holiday shopping and the special gifts you give yourself! If you are trying to match a color, pick up some paint color chips at your local hardware store, make notes on the back of each, and carry them along. Brainstorm gift ideas with the whole family.

- Make maps a part of your trip. Show your children a map before you leave home, and then follow along your route each day. You may be able to find maps in travel brochures that can be added to your scrapbooks.

- Bring a favorite toy. Something from home can bring special comfort to travelers. In addition, a toy can be an amusing character in the story and photos of your trip.

- Look for funny signs. Try to find signs with your children's names or favorite animals on them and take photos.

- Go on a treasure hunt. Choose one item each day and then see how many you can find. For example, how many different elephants (or bridges, or trains) can you find in a day if you include signs, pictures, and toys? Give prizes for the best treasure hunter.

- Learn a word. Pick a new word—in English or in another language—each day and add it to your vocabulary. Try to find a word that's related to what you are seeing—perhaps something in the local geography or architecture. Have everyone practice using it (and write it in their logs).

- Discover something. Each day, have everyone look for something they have never seen before. Talk about it and add it to your daily logs. Notice how plants and animals are different from the ones at home. Do the birds sound different? Are the constellations different from the ones you usually see?

- Review each day. When everyone is together at the end of each day, spend some time talking about what you did, saw, and learned that day. What was strange, scary, or funny? What was the best and worst food? Which things would you do again if you could?

To sum up, begin your intensive planning as soon as the trip becomes a possibility. Starting early allows you to research and prepare thoroughly, not only for fun but also for the safety of you and your children. Plus, your planning will add immeasurably to the joys of anticipation.

The more you prepare for a safe and healthy trip, the more likely you are to have a great time and avoid problems. If you are thoughtful and realistic about your travel plans and expectations, you are sure to have many worthwhile and enjoyable trips with your children.

Chapter 2
Parents' Guide to Safety at Home and Abroad

You dream, you plan, you pack, you go. But how can you keep your family safe as you enjoy your long-awaited and hard-earned vacation? This chapter touches on some of the complex safety issues in today's world—both at home and abroad.

As you read this chapter, visualize yourself in situations where one of these recommendations could save your life or the lives of your children. If you do that mental exercise, you will react more quickly and more effectively if emergency strikes.

Take Care of Yourself First

Parents traveling with children should memorize these important words:

In an emergency, I must take care of myself first so I'll be able to help and protect my children. I'm useless as a parent if I'm unconscious or too badly injured to do what has to be done for them.

The airlines have it right. If the oxygen masks drop, put your own on first, then help your child.

When It Is Just You and Your Child

When adults travel with a child, they are slightly more vulnerable to criminal attack than if they were by themselves. A woman traveling with two or more children is significantly more vulnerable. When you arrive in any country where you will be on less-traveled routes, take the time to meet with consular officials. They will probably be able to offer valuable advice.

Before confirming arrangements for your trip, plan ahead to avoid dangerous places and situations. A woman traveling alone with a child not only needs to be on her guard in airports and public spaces, she also needs to pick safe lodgings. Do not stay in places lacking telephones in the rooms unless you have a working cell phone for that locality. If you need to call the police in the night because someone is trying to break in, the pay phone in the lobby will not help.

The Automobile Club of America recommends that rooms be equipped with a primary lock, to which guests have a key, and a secondary dead bolt that is locked from the inside. This is a far more secure arrangement than a chain, which can easily be cut from the outside. And never leave your hotel door unlocked, even for a moment. Always carry your key and make sure the door locks behind you when you leave. Conceal your room number, and do not write your name on a room service order you hang on your doorknob for pickup.

It's a good idea to provide your child with an identification tag that lists your home phone number and can be worn on a necklace concealed beneath clothing. Also, try to find out about emergency medical facilities in your destination and ask your pediatrician if he or she can recommend a doctor in that area.

Insurance

There are various types of insurance worth considering for your trip: health, auto, medical evacuation, luggage loss/damage, hotel overbooking, and trip cancellation and interruption insurance. Consider obtaining medical evacuation insurance if any member of your party has a chronic health problem or if you will be visiting countries where medical facilities may be far below U.S. standards.

Your decision to purchase travel insurance will be influenced by your destination and the policy terms of your current health, auto, home-owners', and even credit card coverage. Never assume that your current policy will cover you on your trip—it could end up being a very costly assumption.

Shop around for insurance. Most travel policies cost about 5 percent to 7 percent of the cost of the trip. Look for policies that cover your needs, not just for those with the lowest prices. Make sure the policy you are purchasing covers the country you are visiting and the problems that could occur. Read the fine print and make sure you understand the exclusions. Speak with your insurance agent or visit some of the on-line insurance sites listed in Appendix C.

Finding Medical Help Away from Home

As you prepare for your trip, whether you will be staying in the United States or going abroad, ask your internist, pediatrician, or other specialist whether he or she can recommend a physician in your destination. Look for listings of physicians who are certified by the boards of their specialties, such as orthopedics and pediatrics. Or, consult the offices or Internet sites for national associations that represent individual medical conditions (for example, diabetes, multiple sclerosis).

The International Society of Travel Medicine (ISTM) has more than 1,600 members in more than seventy countries. It is the world's largest organization of professionals dedicated to the advancement of travel medicine. Its *Directory of Travel Medicine Clinics and Providers* can be accessed at www.istm.org.

Also check www.highwaytohealth.com for additional information about the countries you select. If you carry a laptop on your trip, you may be able to access a map showing where the nearest English-speaking doctor can be found in the foreign city where you need medical care.

The local U.S. Consulate can probably direct you to the nearest English-speaking doctor, but its hours may be limited.

MedicAlert

If anyone in your family has a serious allergy or medical condition that could make emergency treatment dangerous if unknown to emergency room personnel, consider becoming a member of MedicAlert. For modest fees, this nonprofit organization will provide a wearable emblem that is recognized by doctors and emergency responders worldwide and informs them that the individual's medical records are instantly available on MedicAlert's twenty-four-hour hot line. See Appendix C for contact information and additional details.

Proving Your Child Is Yours

Unless both parents are traveling with the child(ren), and the family is obviously of the same race or nationality, you may have difficulty entering or leaving some countries. Concerns about international child abduction have led many governments to set up preventive procedures at entry and exit points. These often include requiring: (a) documentary evidence of relationship, and (b) if both parents are not present, permission from the nontraveling parent or legal guardian for the child to travel.

Make a color photocopy of the first two pages of both parents' passports (they'll fit on a single sheet of copy paper). This will show both signatures. The absent parent should write, sign, and date a brief letter addressed "To Whom It May Concern" stating that he or she is the father or mother of the named child, and that the traveling parent has his or her permission to take the child from the United States to anywhere in the world or to and from named continents or nations. The travel dates covered by the permission should be stated. Either specify a short period, "between August 1, 2004 and August 20, 2004" or a longer period, such as "at any time" or "from the date of this letter until December 31, 2004."

If a parent traveling with a child cannot follow the above procedures for reasons such as the spouse's death or estrangement, he or she should carry the best documentation obtainable. This might be a certified copy of the other parent's death certificate or custody papers in a divorce situation.

If possible, obtain a passport for the child. Be sure to start this process early. Allow at least six weeks to obtain your child's passport if you foresee no difficulties (as when both parents are available to sign the application); otherwise allow more time.

Such documentation, even if not required, may facilitate entry and departure. This is especially important where an adopted child is of a different race or appears to be from a different background or nation than the adoptive parents. If your children do not have their own passports, carry copies of their birth certificates.

A photograph of the child with the parents may be sufficient in many instances if there are questions or if the child is lost. Carry a current family photo at all times.

Lost Child!

Very few things are as terrifying as suddenly realizing that your child cannot be found. Children seven and younger are especially adventuresome and may not understand the rules to follow when on an outing with family or friends. These rules are simple. Always:

- Keep children in sight.

- Assign an adult to keep track of each child and pair children in the buddy system, older child with younger child.

- Accompany a child to the rest room.

- Make sure a child is not left alone for any reason.

- Choose a conspicuous meeting place and give your children instructions on what to do if they get separated from you.

- Show them police officers or security guards to whom they can go if they get separated from you.

- In large groups, make head-counting an important ritual.

- Carry a current photo of your child.

It is easy for small children to get turned around and disoriented. They can get distracted by something interesting, turn around to look for Mommy, and set out in the wrong direction to find her.

It is especially important to set strict boundaries when you are camping, hiking, or visiting unfamiliar places. Attaching a whistle to each child and teaching them simple signals will make them more responsible and independent while allowing them greater freedom of movement. Handheld two-way radios and cell phones work well for slightly older children.

Depending on his or her age, a wrist handholder or a harness with lead may help you keep track of a difficult child.

Avoiding Abduction

We gaze in horror at the photo of a lost child. Our hearts ache for the desperate parents. We wonder how a child can just disappear. . . . what could the parents have done to prevent it. . . . what could we do to protect our children. For many parents, the thought of having a child taken from them is too terrifying to contemplate. The most dangerous thing, though, is to put the possibility out of your mind. Instead, mentally prepare yourself to lessen the chance— even though it is actually an extremely small one—that one of your children could be abducted.

When you are traveling, do not get so involved in sightseeing that you forget about personal safety. Be aware of the possibility that a criminal can victimize you or someone in your party. In many places, Americans are perceived as fabulously wealthy and easy targets for crime. Also, avoid taking your children to places where anti-American sentiment could make you more vulnerable to crime or attack.

In addition, be sure to always keep your children close to you and keep your family together as much as possible. Tell your children what to do if you get separated, and keep reviewing this instruction with them as your situation changes. Above all, make certain that they—and you—will remain calm if separated. Being lost is not the same as being abducted.

Finally, trust your intuition. If someone who gives you a bad feeling approaches your party, everybody should be trained to move on when the designated leader gives the signal. Make sure that everyone in your travel party understands this tactic, or someone is likely to be left behind.

Abductions do happen. They happen in small towns and big cities, during the day and at night. Yet parents of abducted children always say, "we never would have imagined that it could happen to our family." Here's a list of things you can do that will minimize the chances of your children being abducted or harmed:

1. Educate children early—even before preschool—regarding appropriate behavior toward strangers. Safety skills include not taking anything (such as candy) from a stranger or petting a stranger's puppy. Establish a family code word and teach your children never to go anywhere with someone who doesn't know it.

2. Be aware. Parents, relatives, nannies, and baby-sitters need to be vigilant to be safe. Look around. Be especially alert if you have more than one child, especially twins or triplets.

3. Do not make slightly older siblings responsible for the safety of younger ones; they are only companions who can help reinforce your instructions.

4. If you hire a baby-sitter or nanny, check his or her references carefully and be sure your instructions are clear and well understood before you leave home.

5. Public places, including parks, movie theaters, arcades, stairwells, basements, malls, and parking structures are common places for abductions. Never leave your child unattended.

6. Teach children how to dial 911 and what to say. Make sure they know important names and addresses.

7. Help your children to feel empowered, not terrified. Show them where they can go if they need help (a neighbor's house, police station, church, etc.). Help them to recognize authorities who can assist them, such as police. Teach them they have the right to say "No," to question a stranger's authority, and to scream and scratch to protect themselves from harm.

8. Communicate openly with your children and encourage them to talk with you about their activities, friends, concerns, and plans.

9. Do not advertise your child's name on clothing, bicycles, or backpacks. Abductors may gain a child's trust by calling him or her by name.

10. Teach your children door and phone rules for home and hotel: They should never open the door to a stranger—no matter what that person may say— and they should never tell an unknown caller that you are not at home.

11. Instruct your children to avoid playing or taking shortcuts through abandoned buildings or fields, and make sure they understand the dangers of hitchhiking.

12. Abductors may try to win a child's trust by asking the child to keep a secret or to help find a lost pet. Be sure your child recognizes this danger.

13. Make a meeting plan for public places so your children know what to do if you should get separated at the mall (for example, go to the nearest cashier) or elsewhere (for example, stay in one place and let me find you).

14. Some children first "meet" their abductors on-line. Examine carefully your child's on-line activities and friendships. You may need to help your child

understand that this is an important part of the care you give them and that, until they are eighteen, it is both legally and emotionally more important than their privacy.

15. If you notice a change in your child's behavior, talk with him or her about it. If your child brings home unexplained money or gifts, question him or her carefully.

16. When you are traveling in unfamiliar places or busy with your shopping or cell phone, you may be momentarily distracted and lose track of your child. It takes effort to maintain vigilance.

17. Take notice of people who show an unusual amount of interest in your child.

18. Find out from local law enforcement whether a registered sex offender lives in your community.

19. Keep information about your child current: Take photos at least once a year, more often for preschool age children. Maintain fingerprints, footprints, dental and medical information, birth certificates, and descriptions or photos of birthmarks.

You and your children should be aware and prepared, but you need not live in fear. The more positive communication and coping skills you teach your children, the safer and more comfortable you all will be.

Guarding Against Crime

No one can tell you how to avoid being victimized by every sort of criminal in every possible situation. What follows are some pointers for parents who travel with children. They will help you avoid the most common and dangerous crimes inflicted on travelers.

Shun Dangerous Locales

We take many things for granted when we travel in our own country—political stability, safe drinking water out of the tap, good roads, readily available medical care, well-built hotels, and dependable telephone service. However, things can be much different beyond our shores.

Political violence is constant in some nations. In others, rebellions, violent strikes, and widespread civic unrest and rioting can erupt at any time. You can study current conditions worldwide by accessing the State Department's travel warnings, consular information sheets, and public announcements at www.travel.state.gov/travel_warnings.html, by phone at (202) 647–5225, or by automated telefax at (202) 647–3000.

Be Personally Aware

It is not unusual to take some risks while traveling, such as nighttime sightseeing in unfamiliar places. Make common sense precautions part of your routine. Here are some tips to increase your level of awareness and your safety:

- When using a public rest room stall, do not hang your purse or pocketbook on the door hook where it can be grabbed from outside, over the top of the door.

- Snap a rubber band or two around your wallet. This makes it harder for a pickpocket to remove the wallet unnoticed.

- When you use a telephone charge card, strangers can copy your identification number by watching what numbers you press or by listening to the tones. If possible, use a phone that allows you to swipe your card rather than press numbers.

- You cannot always rely on hotel safes to protect your valuables. Hotels have very limited liability for items left in the hotel safe-deposit vault. Make sure your home-owners' insurance or a separate floater covers valuables left in a hotel vault.

- Use your office address on your luggage identification tags. This way you avoid advertising that your home is vacant.

Avoid Victimization

Travelers tend to be distracted, a bit uncertain, and in a hurry to make connections—all things that make them easier targets for criminals. These tips will lessen your chances of becoming a victim:

- Avoid traveling on public transport during rush hours. Be particularly careful when in dense crowds, while standing in line, or while getting on or off trains, buses, or aircraft. Traveling with a group provides greater security.

- Use only labeled taxis, even if someone offers a "deal."

- Rely on the hotel concierge to arrange for theater tickets, cabs, tours, restaurant reservations, and other needs.

- Carry your own luggage, if possible, and do not let it out of your sight. Keep your purse or wallet with you at all times.

- For added protection, carry a whistle to attract attention or a personal alarm that shrieks if activated.

- Obtain a readable street map of every city you plan to visit. Memorize map routes in your hotel room or while in a restaurant so that you do not have to study them as you walk.

- When out for a stroll, make it look like you know where you are going. Try to look more like a native and not advertise that you are a tourist. Walk with purpose, especially if you are alone.

- If you are a victim of crime, report it to the police as soon as possible, as most insurance claims require a police report.

Stow Your Valuables

While you are focused on the scenery, you—and your belongings—may be the focus of thieves. Ever more devious in their deceptions, street thugs make off every day with cash, wallets, purses, suitcases, jewelry, cameras, watches, and other valuables they have pilfered from tourists. And although we would like to think these things happen only "after dark" in "bad neighborhoods" or in "other countries," they can happen any time of day and anywhere people fail to be vigilant.

Where common sense used to be enough to protect you, today you need to stay one step ahead of the criminals. As you prepare for your trip, consider the following:

- Carry as little as possible.

- Leave valuable jewelry and watches, expensive shoes, and leather jackets at home. Rule of thumb regarding a possession: If you would be extremely unhappy to lose it, do not take it.

- Eliminate the extraneous bulk from your wallet—or eliminate your wallet altogether. Stash some small notes for taxi rides and purchases in buttoned pockets, but keep the bulk of your money and your passport in a security pouch concealed beneath your clothing. (Relocate your valuables to waist, thigh, or shoe if you plan to wear open-necked clothing that will reveal the strap of your neck pouch.)

- Women should carry purses with a substantial shoulder strap and wear the purse across the body rather than hanging from the shoulder. If you are wearing an outer coat, put the coat on over your purse. If you carry a purse, choose one that has a zippered top with a flap over it and turn it so that it faces your body.

- Do not rely on the security of fanny packs, backpacks, or shoulder bags. Thieves can slash or grab and be gone before you know what has happened. Be especially vigilant in restaurants; setting something on the floor beside your chair is an open invitation to thievery.

- When you go shopping, do not load yourself down with packages.

- Always let someone know where you are going and when you will return.

- Carry as few credit cards as possible. Before you leave home, make a list of your credit card numbers and leave it with someone who can cancel them at your request should they become lost or stolen.

- Leave a record of your itinerary, your traveler's checks serial numbers, and photocopies of your air tickets and the identifying pages of your passport at home with a friend in case any of these items are lost or stolen while you are traveling.

- Keep an up-to-date list of your traveler's checks, carried separately from the checks themselves.

In a recent issue of *Condé Nast Traveler*, travel magazine columnist Wendy Perrin reported on a number of scams designed to distract tourists and make them ripe for picking by waiting thieves, including these ploys:

- Spraying, splashing, or spilling something on you, quickly followed by "helpful" gestures, all in the hope that you will put down whatever you are carrying.

- Staged fights followed by a plea for money to get to the doctor—an effort to get your wallet out of your pocket.

- Various ATM scams, with "helpful" thieves standing by.

- Crowd action, wherein a group of people, including very small children, causes a diversion in a subway car or street crowd as others relieve people of their valuables.

- Car scams, such as tire slashings, bogus parking attendants, or even fake accidents designed to give thieves access to your possessions.

- Airport screening scams, which easily separate people from their valuables as the passenger ahead sets off the alarm.

- The nefarious "baby toss," with someone hurriedly handing off a child (or even a doll), hoping that the unsuspecting tourist will drop his or her bags.

Being aware of some of the treachery that is designed for tourists can help you to get ready both physically and mentally. Prepare yourself for your travels. Do your homework on your destination. Pack light. Once there, look around. Stay alert. Use common sense. Trust your intuition.

Child-Friendly Hotel Rooms

Staying in a hotel can be an exciting part of a family travel adventure for everyone. Before you turn in for the night, take a few minutes to examine the facilities, talk about the rules, and assure yourself that your children will be as safe in the hotel as they are at home.

Hotel Room Safety Checklist

1. Review all safety and ground rules upon arrival.

2. Discuss never opening the door to a stranger. Discuss room service procedure.

3. Be aware that with that extra room for children, a hotel may also be providing potentially dangerous equipment such as refrigerator, stove, and cooking utensils.

4. Be sure medications, soaps, cleaners, and liquor are high overhead and safe.

5. Consider hiring a professional baby-sitter, even if you are in the next room.

6. Be sure all rooms are safe. Check locks on all windows and doors.

7. Review the location of emergency exits and make sure smoke detectors are working. Also count the number of doors you must pass to get to the emergency exit or stairwell. Fire safety review is a must.

8. Instruct children to keep luggage off the floor; falling over luggage can be dangerous at any age. Also remember that your luggage, packed with medications and other supplies and equipment, could be tempting and dangerous to a curious toddler. Keep it locked and out of reach.

9. Review television and telephone limitations and adjust them as appropriate.

10. Pack a plug-in night-light for the bathroom. Finding the bathroom in a strange place in the middle of the night can be tricky.

11. Many hotels have swimming pools and spas, so be sure to discuss water safety. (There is some risk of infection in hot tubs, especially when children in diapers have been using them. Avoid hot pools if you have open cuts, and always shower with soap and water after getting out of the pool.)

12. Walk around the hotel grounds and point out geographic landmarks and hazards, such as driveways. Decide on a meeting place outside your hotel room in case you should get separated.

As you are exploring the hotel and reviewing the rules, look the room over and make sure it looks freshly cleaned and ready for occupancy. The towels should look and smell clean; the bed linens should be crisp and fresh. The wastebaskets, tub, shower, sinks, and drawers should be free of used soap, tissues, bandages, hair, and other items that show less than diligent cleaning. If you are not satisfied with the cleanliness of the room, request that the room be re-cleaned or that you be moved to an acceptable room. If the hotel is not able to accommodate your needs, find another place to stay.

Family Fire Safety

With our smoke detectors, fire drills, and rules against playing with matches and smoking in bed, most of us feel modestly safe at home. But when we venture away from home, our protection against fire is more likely to depend upon awareness and wits than on standard safety measures. This is especially true in hotels, where an assortment of strangers sleep under the same roof, and you have no way of knowing whether one of them will start a fire. Here are several ways to help you increase your family's chances of surviving a hotel fire:

1. Select where you will stay with an eye to fire safety. Choose two-story or three-story hotels instead of higher buildings, if you have a choice. Fire-truck ladders only reach to about the seventh floor. Do not take a room that is higher. Get a room on the street side that is most readily accessible to fire trucks.

2. Determine your best route out of the building. Do this before you unpack. Go out into the hall and reconnoiter your escape routes. There should be two exits from your floor; check them both in case your first choice is blocked when you need it. As you check on your two exits, visualize finding them when the corridor is pitch black. Get it firmly fixed in your mind whether you should turn left or right when you leave your room. If you find a fire exit padlocked, report it to the management and the fire department and do not accept the room until the exit is cleared.

3. Prepare mentally to cope with an emergency. Make sure everyone understands that in case of fire, everything not living gets left behind. Mentally rehearse how you will lead your family to safety through dark, smoke-filled corridors.

4. Organize for quick departure. Put a flashlight beside your bed along with your room key, your credit cards, money, and passport if you are outside

the United States. Put these things in a security pouch you can pull on quickly so your hands will be free in case you have to crawl.

5. Plan your exit tactics. Touch the door and the doorknob with the back of your hand to check for heat. Get on your knees before you open the door a crack to peek out. If there is smoke but no fire in the hall, reach up with your hand and see if the air higher up is noticeably hotter. If it is not, stand up slowly and check the air temperature. If the air is cool, grab outer clothing and lead your family quickly to the exit. If the hall is very hot but not on fire, lead your family on a fast crawl to the exit.

6. If there is fire in the hall, prepare to lead your family through fire to safety. Protect each person with multiple layers of clothes, blankets, towels, pillows, and seat cushions; these will protect you from heat for a short period and will protect you from flames momentarily. Cloth will catch on fire but can be discarded as you go. Stay close to the wall.

7. When you reach the emergency exit, proceed slowly down the stairs. Never get in an elevator when there is a fire in the building.

8. If fire traps you in your room, use wet sheets and blankets to block cracks around the doors and windows and stop smoke from entering the room. Give the fire department time to rescue you.

9. Increase your family's safety with simple technology. Consider adding flashlights, a portable smoke alarm, fire resistant gloves and goggles, and a cell phone to your travel kit.

Hazards at Holiday Time

Unfortunately, some of our most important holidays involve special risks of injury. Since family travel is often associated with holidays, some of the most common concerns are listed here.

It does not take much alcohol to poison children because their bodies are small; amounts that would make an adult merely tipsy can be extremely dangerous if consumed by a child. The day after a party, some children who wake early might think it fun to explore the party room and sample what is left in glasses, or even light up cigarettes—fresh ones if cigarette packages are lying around, butts if ashtrays are overflowing. This means it is important to clean up before going to bed, which is easily done if the party is held in your own home. However, if you and your children travel to spend the night with friends at the party house, you may want to discuss the matter with your hosts before agreeing to attend, or leave your children at home with a baby-sitter.

Fourth of July

Injuries from fireworks have been on a downward trend for many years, but several thousand children are still being injured by fireworks every year in the United States. Use caution on this holiday. Close adult supervision of children is essential, even with legal fireworks. Do not permit young children to use fireworks. Under no circumstances should guns be fired into the air; bullets fired into the air injure and kill people on their way down.

Many communities have professional fireworks displays. It is wise and more fun to take the family to these public displays rather than risk injury by using fireworks at home.

Halloween

Every Halloween, the media reports cases in which trick-or-treating children come to harm. Responsible adults must accompany children on these excursions. Better yet, some communities and organizations offer indoor Halloween programs to replace the house-to-house activities. Find out what your community or the community you are visiting has to offer.

Any time a person wears a mask, such as on Halloween, Mardi Gras, or New Year's Eve, there is a risk of impaired vision. Because adults often wear masks on these occasions, children may not recognize them and may be more easily drawn away from the group. Children are especially at risk when they are trick-or-treating, crossing streets, and moving around in the dark.

Parents should inspect everything that children bring home on Halloween and throw out anything that offers the slightest suspicion of danger. Adult supervision is absolutely required in any children's activities and especially those at Halloween.

Thanksgiving

This uniquely American holiday is a traditional time for family gatherings. For many the greatest hazard of this holiday is the automobile journey. If you can, leave early enough to be at your destination on Wednesday, ahead of the throng of travelers.

If you have little ones who tend to poke at everything, pop anything in their mouths—if they do not stuff it up their noses—and pull anything—no matter how heavy or hot—down on themselves, you have a serious problem to solve when going to the homes of relatives or friends. You have three choices:

1. Keep your little one on your lap at all times.

2. Use a restraining harness with lead to prevent your child from roaming.

3. Childproof the house you are visiting.

Christmas

All the concerns of Thanksgiving also apply at Christmas. In addition you are likely to encounter poisonous plants inside the home during this season. Mistletoes and holly berries are known to be gastric irritants that cause stomach aches, or worse, even when just a few berries are ingested by younger children. Be careful to pick up any leaves or berries as soon as they fall from these plants so they can be kept from the eager hands and mouths of curious children. Even if they don't cause poisoning, these small objects can be a choking hazard. Remember, children and pets are much smaller and are affected by a much smaller quantity if the plant is ingested.

Decorated Christmas trees, with their strings of electric lights and delicate glass ornaments, can be an irresistible pull-down hazard to a toddler or small child. Snow sprays contain solvents and should be used according to directions in well-ventilated rooms, though they are considered safe once dry. Broken decorations, such as bubble lights and glass balls, can be dangerous if ingested. Tinsel and icicles may be choking hazards. And the wrappings and holiday ribbons decorated with small, bright objects may intrigue very small children more than the gifts themselves. After gifts have been unwrapped, make sure there are no baubles—or small batteries!—left lying around that fit into little mouths or noses.

Holiday times are for enjoyment. By taking adequate precautions and keeping careful watch on your children, your holidays and theirs will be filled with excitement and result in long-lasting, happy memories.

The Poisons Around Us

The world can be a toxic place for curious children. They can be poisoned by swallowing substances, spilling or splashing them on the skin or in the eyes, getting stung or bitten, or breathing toxic fumes. Although just a few minutes of care could remove many of these hazards from the home, children are most commonly poisoned by cleaning products, pesticides, drugs and medications, cosmetics, plants, paints, and solvents.

Children who are not supervised are the ones most likely to find their way into bathroom drawers or medicine cabinets or "under the sink"—places filled with danger to probing youngsters. In fact, late afternoon, when many children find themselves unsupervised, is called the "arsenic hour" at poison centers.

Even if you carefully monitor toxic substances in your home, a visit to friends or relatives, an afternoon at the baby-sitter's, a stay in a vacation rental or campground, or a few minutes with a guest's handbag could put your child at risk.

If your child is poisoned, call 911 (in the United States) or other knowledgeable help immediately. If there is time, call your pediatrician or the local poison center. To locate the poison center nearest you, look in your telephone directory or call (202) 362–7217. Post these emergency numbers next to every telephone in your house and add local numbers to your phone list when you travel.

Swallowing poison is the most common danger. If you suspect that a child has swallowed poison, make the child spit it out or remove it with a swipe of your fingers. Do not make the child vomit; strong acids and alkalis can damage the throat and mouth.

Look for the following symptoms of poisoning and tell the paramedics or poison center if you observe any of them:

- stomach cramps without fever or nausea

- burns on the lips or mouth

- severe throat pain

- difficulty breathing

- unusual behavior, drooling, odor, or clothing stains

Do not forget that liquor can be poisonous to small children. Keep it locked up.

If a harmful substance is *spilled or splashed* on your child, remove the child's clothing and rinse the area with lukewarm—not hot—water for about fifteen minutes, even if the child resists. Do not use oil, grease, or ointments. Call the poison center and follow the advice given.

If the *substance is in the eye*, wash the eye by holding the eyelid open and pouring a steady stream of lukewarm water into the inner corner of the eye. If necessary, have someone hold the child for you. If you are alone, wrap the child tightly in a towel, clamp him or her under your arm, and use both hands to wash the eye.

Poisonous fumes can occur anywhere: car exhaust in a closed space, leaky gas appliances, defective wood, coal or oil stoves, or aerosol inhalants. Get the child into fresh air immediately. If the child is breathing, call the poison center. If not, begin CPR until breathing is restarted or someone can relieve you. Have someone call 911. If you are alone, call 911 after breathing is restarted or after one minute of CPR.

Stings and bites are sources of poisoning from insects, spiders, scorpions, and snakes. Because of their small size, children can be affected more seriously by such toxins than are adults. Allergies or reactions to stings can be life threatening. Before going on a trip, check with your pediatrician and be sure to take along the appropriate medication if your child has known allergies. If your child is bitten by a snake, treat it as a serious poisoning. Keep the child calm and call the poison center or 911. Follow the instructions you're given exactly. If you are unable to call, follow the directions in your snakebite kit.

Do not rely on the instructions about poisoning found on package labels; they may be outdated and no longer helpful in light of modern research. Take the poison away from the child and keep the container for reference. Stay calm. Follow exactly the instructions you get from the paramedics or the poison center.

If you suspect poisoning—by swallowing, spilling or inhaling, or by an insect, spider, or snakebite—call the poison center even if the child does not have any symptoms. Provide as much information as possible, reading from package labels where available and responding to the advisor's questions. Most children are not permanently harmed by poisons if they are treated right away. Prevention and observation are the best ways to avoid poisoning—at home and on the road.

Childproofing Checklist

Childproof your own home first. Doing this will make you an expert childproofer so you can quickly spot—and eliminate or guard against—the greatest dangers when visiting with your children in someone else's home or at hotels, campgrounds, and other facilities.

Bathrooms

- Make sure no electrical devices such as clocks, radios, TVs, and hair dryers could fall or be pulled down into the tub or sink.

- When medicines are no longer used, flush the remainder away.

- Small children imitate. Avoid taking medicine in front of them.

- When giving a child medication, check the label every time to make sure you are giving the right dose of the right medicine. Dangerous mistakes of this kind are most often made at night, so be extra careful when you get up from a sound sleep. Do not hurry; turn on a light; make sure you are doing the right thing.

- Never tell a child that medicine is candy to get them to take it; this plants dangerous ideas in their heads.

- Store the most commonly used items—soap, shampoo, toothpaste, and so on—away from dangerous products, which should be kept in a locked cabinet.

- If you visit homes where young children are not present most of the time, look for containers that a curious child can easily open. Bear in mind that child-*resistant* containers are not child*proof*.

Kitchen

- Dangerous household products—such as drain cleaner, bleach, lye, furniture polish, and dishwasher soap—are often kept under the sink. If so, secure the doors with a padlock.

- One of the greatest dangers to small children is their tendency to pull things down on themselves. Serious burns result if your child pulls something hot down from the stove. Either keep the little ones out of the kitchen by installing a gate, or do your cooking in a microwave oven.

- Never use soft drink bottles or other food or drink containers to store dangerous products.

- Make sure that kitchen drawers have stops so they can't be pulled all the way out on top of a curious child.

- Store sharp knives in a locked cabinet or drawer.

Living Room

- Cords that hang down where a crawling child can reach them are dangerous for two reasons: (1) Children can pull clocks, telephones, computers, and other equipment down on themselves and sustain a severe injury. (2) Small ones can get entangled in the cords and strangle.

- Unprotected electrical outlets invite curious little people to poke something into those intriguing holes to see what will happen. The result could be serious.

- Women's handbags are likely to be put on the living room floor where a child can get into them. Some of those purses may contain medications that could be lethal to a small child.

- Never leave a child unattended in a room when a fire is burning in the fireplace.

Basement or Garage Storage Area

If you keep paint, thinners, pesticides, power tools, sharp tools of all kinds, and machinery in a separate locked building, you have this problem under control.

However, it is common for such things to be stored in a basement or garage, where your children are more likely to get into trouble with them. With careful consideration, these risks can be minimized.

- Dangerous tools and substances must be kept in locked cabinets.

- Before you buy household products, study the labels. Choose the least-toxic brands and buy no more than you can use immediately.

- Paint and similar products are often kept on dusty shelves when they can no longer be used. When you buy paint, note the date it should be thrown away on the lid. A can of paint too old to be used can be as much of a fire hazard as is fresh paint.

- Make sure that sharp tools—especially power tools and machinery—are kept under lock and key.

Firearms

Whether they are collectors, hunters, or just concerned about personal safety, many people have guns in the home and many people carry firearms when they travel. Guns in the home are more than forty times more likely to be used in the killing of a friend or family member than in self-defense. Many firearm deaths and injuries, accidental or intentional, involve children—as either victims or perpetrators. Whatever your attitude about guns, if you have both guns and children in your home, you must keep your firearms locked up securely and teach children about gun safety.

- Remove ammunition from guns and store guns and ammunition separately.

- Keep guns and ammunition under lock and key and do not allow children access to the key.

- Teach children that *guns are not toys*. They are deadly weapons. Emphasize that the fantasy of violence and death that they may see on television or in movies is not real ("dead" people on TV often show up alive in another program).

- If you are going on a backcountry hiking or hunting trip and will be carrying a gun, do not ever leave children unattended around firearms.

- Remember that small, curious children can easily discover guns "hidden" in drawers, suitcases, glove boxes, closets, and pockets.

- If you are visiting friends or family, make sure they are diligent about firearm safety as well.

- Repeat gun safety training regularly as children mature to increase their chances of living safe and healthy lives.

Safe and Healthy Play Places

More than a quarter of a million children fifteen years or younger each year are injured and treated in emergency rooms for playground-related incidents. Playgrounds, homes, fast-food restaurants, and resorts have various types of play equipment for children. Although manufacturing standards, building and safety rules, and school regulations govern nearly all of the play places in the United States, this may not be true in other places you visit. Older play equipment may be ignored and it can become hazardous.

Check all play equipment for safety, especially if it appears old or worn. Do not rely on someone else to be as thorough as necessary to protect your children from danger.

Begin your inspection at the play area fence, which should be free of sharp wires and splinters. Look for guardrails around raised platforms and make sure steps have rails. Watch for spaces that could trap a curious child's head; openings in equipment should be either fewer than 3½ inches wide or more than 9 inches wide.

Playground Surface

Luxuriantly thick grass is probably the best surface for under home-play equipment, but it may conceal rocks or sprinkler heads that are trip-and-fall hazards.

If the surface under equipment is sand or wood chips, it should be 10 to 12 inches deep. The protective material should be clean, not loaded with animal droppings or dirt. The concrete footings of the equipment should not protrude above the surface. Check footings for jagged edges that can cause injuries.

At many parks and schools, the protective surface is inch-thick rubberized material laid over blacktop. Look for exposed blacktop where the rubber has worn away.

The safe surface area should extend well beyond the footing of play equipment. For slides and climbing equipment, it should extend at least 4 feet beyond the equipment. Swings should have a clear area all the way around equal to twice the swing's height.

Backyard playgrounds often have too little space for the equipment installed in them, raising the risk of children falling onto rocks, sprinkler heads, or other hard things crowding the play space. Child care centers may have more play equipment than the available space can safely accommodate.

Slides

Check the slide bed for sharp points that can slice a leg or hand open as a child slides over it. Before allowing your children onto a slide in hot weather, or any time their legs are bare, run your hand over every part of the sliding surface that is, or has been, in direct sunlight. Watch for dangerous handrails on the top platform of the slide. Some of them can catch little arms and pitch the sliders over the side. Look for slide ladder handles coming to a sharp V that can cause injuries if hands or arms get caught in the V.

Make sure of three things before allowing your child to use a slide:

1. The bottom of the slide should be the right height for children to get their feet under them when they reach the bottom, so they will not get thrown off on their backs.

2. If the landing place is a hole pounded in the earth by thousands of landings, sprinklers or rain can turn this hole into mud. Dry or muddy, the hole is an easy place to twist an ankle.

3. Retaining walls, rocks, sprinkler heads, and other hazards should be far enough away so a child coming off the slide will not be pitched onto them.

Swings

Oblong holes under swings and slide exits indicate that the equipment has not recently been examined or maintained. Another obvious sign of neglect is that the equipment squeaks when it is being used. On swings, this indicates rapid wear on swing bearings. On other equipment, it may indicate loose parts or weak parts that may break at any time.

Look at the links of chain at the top where wear is greatest. If any link is halfway worn through, the entire chain must be replaced before further use. Many backyard swings have no bearings so that the top link of the chain grinds against a metal hook. Rapid wear can cause a chain to break.

Homemade swings often use ropes tied to a tree limb instead of chain supported by a steel or wood structure. This may make for a wonderful swing, but the ropes can wear through quickly or saw through the tree limb. Rope and tree swings should be inspected frequently to make sure they are safe.

Bear in mind that at some point during its travel, an unoccupied swing seat, as when a child jumps out of it, will be moving fast at the head height of any toddler who wanders into its path. Do not allow your little one near swing sets.

Swing seats should be made of a light, flexible, rubberized material rather than hard plastic, heavy wood, or any kind of metal. They should also be free of any sharp projections. Children under five years of age should use chair swings.

Trampolines

Trampolines are often found in backyards, at camps, on playgrounds, and in school gyms, and their improper use is the cause of numerous injuries, mainly among children ages four to fourteen. Injuries range from simple sprains to head, neck, and spinal cord damage and broken bones. Even a very small trampoline raised just a few inches off the ground can result in a twisted ankle—or worse. A trampoline should be used for gymnastics or other appropriate sports activities *only under the supervision of a trained professional.*

Climbing Apparatuses of All Kinds

A soft surface—sand, wood chips, or rubber matting—should be provided under climbing equipment. Check equipment and footings for exposed nails, screws, sharp bolts, hooks, sharp edges, and splinters that could cause injuries.

If you see dangerous conditions on a school playground, inform the school principal. If the playground is at a public park, contact the recreation director at city hall. Phone in your report and then follow it up with a written report.

Safety on Wheels

Whether at home, at camp, or on vacation, your children probably entertain themselves with an assortment of wheeled play equipment: tricycles, wagons, scooters, skateboards, roller and in-line skates, and bicycles, among others. Many of these "toys" today are offered in a motorized version, with an unsurprising increase in injuries to their users. Here are a few safety guidelines:

- Make sure that wheels are securely fastened to the equipment and properly inflated.

- Equip children with protective gear, such as helmets, gloves, knee pads, elbow pads, and wrist guards. Remember to be a good model; do not expect your children to wear helmets if they see you riding your bike without one.

- Accompany small children, watch them carefully, and coach them around hazards such as rocks and sidewalk irregularities.

- Carefully explain the hazards of driveways and teach small children to stop and look before riding across a driveway. A child on a tricycle is below the rearview visibility of a driver backing into the street.

- Teach children to use hand signals for slowing/stopping and turning.

- Demonstrate bike etiquette, especially around pedestrians. Not all pedestrians can hear bike bells or horns, and most will be startled by a small person hurtling by at top speed shouting "Look out!"

- As older children graduate from the sidewalk to the road, teach them about the dangers of cars pulling out of parking places and driveways and, very importantly, drivers opening their doors into the bike lane.

- When you travel, check with the local police, auto club, or sporting goods stores to find out whether there are laws or regulations related to wheeled sports and also whether there are designated bike paths, roller rinks, and skateboard zones.

Safety Tips for Various Age Groups

Newborn to Six Months

Obviously, a newborn baby needs constant care.

- Keep baby's face free of obstructions and coverings.

- Check on baby often.

- Check arms, legs, or neck to see if baby is warm enough.

- Make sure you have received feeding instructions.

- Use proper bottle procedures:

    ○ Test temperatures of liquids with a drop or two on the inside of your wrist.

    ○ Cool liquids are fine for infants, but avoid excessively cold liquids.

- Follow these steps when feeding the baby:

    ○ Sit down with the baby.

    ○ Hold the baby firmly, but comfortably, in a semisitting position.

    ○ Do not prop up the bottle; the infant could choke.

    ○ Always support the head and neck when picking up an infant.

    ○ Always burp the baby after feeding. Place the infant in an upright position against the front of your shoulder.

- Be especially careful when bathing an infant because he or she cannot sit up in the tub unaided.

- Never leave the baby on top of anything from which he or she might roll off and fall.

- Keep the baby in the crib with the sides raised when not tending to the child.

- Beware of swallowing hazards, as it is natural for babies to put things in their mouths.

- All potentially hazardous items should be kept up and out of children's reach. Allow a margin of safety; curious children often can reach higher than you think they can.

Six to Twelve Months

During this period, babies will roll over, rock on hands and knees, sit up, start to crawl, and pull themselves up to standing.

- Be alert for dangers to crawlers:
    - lamp and phone cords
    - matches and lighters left on the table
    - electrical outlets
    - cleansers and medications
    - kitchen utensils
    - buckets of water

- Keep the bathroom door securely fastened; a curious baby can drown in a toilet.

- Play simple games such as peekaboo and pat-a-cake with the baby.

- Provide age-appropriate toys:
    - blocks
    - big, brightly colored wooden beads
    - rubber or plastic chewing toys
    - large bells
    - balls
    - pots and pans
    - large wooden spoons
    - large, nontoxic crayons

- Avoid inappropriate toys:
    - older sibling's toys that may present a danger to a younger baby

○ Lego-type building blocks, as they are a choking hazard

○ sharp-edged or pointed toys

○ pencils, pens, and paintbrushes with pointed handles

○ modeling compounds (nontoxic, but a potential choking hazard)

○ breakable things

○ containers that resemble household chemicals and cleansers

○ medicine containers

Twelve to Twenty-four Months

Roaming around the house is normal at this age, but these youngsters require constant supervision.

- Be sure that any safety gates at the top and bottom of stairways are latched.

- Watch out for the child poking things into electrical outlets.

- Make sure the toddler cannot pull things down from the stove, tables, or high shelves.

- Keep common household poisonous substances out of toddler's reach:

  ○ cleansers

  ○ pesticides

  ○ bleach

  ○ aspirin

  ○ motor or machine oils

  ○ paint

  ○ furniture polish

  ○ floor wax

  ○ drain opener

- Don't forget that toddlers can climb. Even cabinets above the floor may be accessible to the child.

- Know the child's favorite toy and keep it handy at nap time.

Two Years

When there is a two-year-old in the house, anything can happen.

- Make sure all doors leading to hazards or outside are securely latched or locked.

- Never take your eyes off a toddler when around water.

- Never let toddlers touch electronics, kitchen appliances, or household machines.

- Always secure the door to the laundry area.

- Latch the door behind you.

- Make sure that all windows are latched or that sufficient window guards are in place.

- Engage children with these activities:

  - puzzles

  - toys that can be taken apart and put back together

  - coloring books

  - stuffed animals

Three Years

The typical three-year-old has finally accomplished some self-control, and he or she is usually cooperative.

- Look out for hazards that might cause a fall. A three-year-old will run—not walk—to do everything.

- Make the child use the handrails on stairways.

- Be careful when outdoors, as the child may dart off without looking.

- Always hold the child's hand when crossing streets and driveways or in parking lots.

- Provide plenty of opportunities for the following activities:

  - picture books

  - peg boards

  - blocks

  - dolls and stuffed animals

- telling stories

- learning simple songs

Four Years

Four-year-olds can be very active.

- Reinforce the rules for riding a tricycle or pedaling a toy car on the sidewalk or your driveway.

- Make sure your child follows the rules about stopping and looking both ways before chasing a ball into the street.

- Always supervise play equipment from which the child may fall or otherwise get injured.

- Reinforce proper playground rules such as walking around, not through, the swing area.

- Keep an eye on older children, especially siblings, who often play too rough for the younger ones.

- Keep a supply of the following on hand:

  - finger paints

  - modeling compound

  - paper and crayons

  - blunt scissors

  - chalkboard

Five to Seven Years

At this age children do not like being treated "like a baby." Most can dress themselves but still may need help with things like shoelaces or zippers.

- Make sure children jump, skip, and turn somersaults in a safe environment.

- Don't let things get out of hand when children play running games, hide and seek, tag, blind man's bluff, and so forth.

- Allow bicycle and skateboard riding only in a safe area, with proper safety equipment.

- Do not allow children to play with sharp sticks, knives, darts, or projectile weapons.

Children and Disaster: Coping with Crisis

Mind-numbing events can happen at home as well as on the road. When disaster strikes, whether it is fire, earthquake, storm, or man-made, children are especially vulnerable and need extra care. Even if you can shelter your children from the visual and auditory assault of televised bad news, they will sense the stress felt by the adults around them.

You may have been directly or indirectly affected by a disaster. You may, in fact, be overwhelmed by emotions and responsibilities in the wake of such an event. As you are swept up in the urgent demands on your time, it is particularly important to ensure that your children get the attention and affection they need so they do not become secondary victims of the disaster.

It is common and normal for children to show feelings and exhibit unusual behavior after a traumatic event. They may revert to behaviors they've outgrown. After a disaster, children may experience any of the following:

- They may fear being alone, being abandoned, or being separated. They may be especially clingy, want to sleep with parents, or resist being alone outside the house or in the bathroom. They may not want to go to school or be left with a baby-sitter.

- Sleep may be disrupted by dreams or nightmares, worry, or bed-wetting.

- Eating and toilet habits may be disrupted.

- Children may be fearful of familiar objects—planes, fire engines, animals— and they may startle at loud noises.

- Children may experience physical complaints such as stomachache or headache.

- Other behavioral changes may include increased apathy, shyness, irritability, aggressiveness, or hyperactivity.

Your children may react immediately or slowly, subtly or dramatically. The sooner you take the time to talk to them, the better. The following suggestions may be helpful; you should anticipate repeating these actions again and again to help your child return to "normal":

- Whatever you may be feeling, give your children your complete attention when you talk with them.

- Encourage your children to discuss their feelings about the disaster. Acknowledge their feelings and let them know that other children are feeling the same thing. Talk about what you are feeling as well.

- Suggest drawing, painting, clay, and toys that may help your children express their fears and concerns where language is inadequate.

- Assure your child that you are safe and together.

- Hold your child and give reassuring touch.

- Talk about what happened in age-appropriate terms that your child can understand.

- Tell children that in a disaster there are many people who can help them.

- Talk about ways that disasters can be prevented or their effects minimized, and empower your children by allowing them to participate in preparations.

- Minimize your child's exposure to television coverage of the disaster.

- Your children may experience actual loss (of family, friend, home, pet, or precious objects) or loss "by proxy" when disasters are physically distant. Allow them to mourn their loss and respect the seriousness of their feelings.

- Encourage your children to take small steps toward mastering their fear. They may need to be slowly desensitized to a feared place or object. Accompany them and talk about how they are getting stronger. Acknowledge and reward their bravery and accomplishments as they move in this direction.

- As conditions return to normal, gently insist upon predisaster behavior. In some cases, a child's unusual behavior may persist, and you may need to seek professional assistance:

  o Regressive behavior lasts more than a few weeks.

  o The child persists in refusing to return to school, eat, or go outside.

  o New symptoms emerge after several weeks.

  o The child's schoolwork shows a significant decline.

  o The child acts out dangerous behavior toward siblings, pets, or self.

Children model much of their behavior on the actions of the adults around them. Your children may be observing you even when you are not paying attention to them. If you are calm and confident and you make an effort to resume the normal patterns of your own life, your children will move more quickly into behavior that will help them cope with the situation.

Chapter 3
Health Guidelines to Follow

Although information about vaccines, prevention methods, and treatment of the most common travelers' problems are included in this chapter, this book is not designed to replace the advice of your physician, pediatrician, family doctor, or travel medicine specialist. Prior to going on any trip, if your child seems sick or has a bothersome temperature, be sure the child is evaluated by your pediatrician, family doctor, or medical facility emergency room. The doctor's evaluation and your "gut feeling" as parents will tell you whether or not to postpone your trip.

Unless it is truly necessary to take very young children to high-risk areas, it may be best not to expose them to malaria, yellow fever, cholera, and other serious diseases. They cannot be protected from some of these diseases, and children are particularly vulnerable to exposure and infection. If your infant shows signs of fever, lethargy, diarrhea, or poor feeding, he or she should be evaluated immediately by a medical professional, even if it means evacuating the child a considerable distance to a proper medical facility.

When you consult with a physician, in person or on the phone, before, during, or after your trip, prepare yourself with the answers to the questions listed in Appendix C. The more detailed and accurate your answers, the quicker he or she will be able to advise you. The research you do before you talk with the physician will help you ask informed questions and improve your understanding of the advice you receive.

Today's travelers can easily obtain updated information about vaccination requirements and infectious disease risks at home and in foreign countries. A visit to the Centers for Disease Control (CDC) Internet site at www.cdc.gov/travel will provide current information and answer vital questions about the regions you plan to visit, such as:

- What are the required and recommended immunizations for all ages, including infants?

- How can I find a travel clinic for immunizations and travel advice for my family's specific needs?

- What are the appropriate disease prevention strategies in my destinations?

- Are there any disease outbreaks or epidemics taking place now in the countries I plan to visit?

- How did my intended cruise ship score in the CDC's reports of its latest sanitary inspection?

Health and safety conditions in the world change rapidly. Check with the CDC for the latest updates any time and any place you plan to travel. If you do not have Internet access in your home, the nearest public library may offer this service, or you can call the CDC's toll-free travelers' health hot line number at (877) FYI–TRIP (394–8747).

Research and development of new vaccines and medicines is ongoing. If your doctor is not knowledgeable in travel medicine, look for a travel medicine specialist or travel clinic. See Appendix C for additional information.

Safe Food and Water

Wherever your travels take you, one of the easiest and most important things you can do to protect your family's health is to establish safe food and water habits. One of the best rules to establish early on whether at home or traveling is to always wash hands—yours and children's—before handling food and after toilet or diapering. If you cannot use soap and water, use a waterless washing solution.

If you are leaving the United States, check for travelers' health alerts in the countries you plan to visit and follow instructions carefully. In remote areas, developing countries, or places where sanitation is questionable, here are some basic safety rules:

- Drink only canned or bottled carbonated beverages, beer, and wine, and hot drinks made with boiled water, such as tea and coffee.

- Before drinking from a bottle or can, wipe the surface that will touch your mouth.

- Avoid ice.

- Do not drink water from bottles or carafes labeled as drinking water; it may be nothing more than tap water. Metal bottle tops can be removed and replaced; they do not ensure the water is safe.

- Do not use tap water to brush your teeth (and keep your mouth shut in the shower!).

- When it comes to food, "Cook it, peel it, or leave it."

- Avoid food that is warm or room temperature or uncooked. Cooked foods should be served hot. In fact, they should be too hot to eat when they reach your table.

- Avoid salads and eat only those fruits and vegetables that are cooked and served hot or can be peeled or shelled. (Avoid those with damaged skin.)

- Never eat raw meat or shellfish and be especially cautious about both raw and cooked fish, which can contain dangerous toxins.

- Be aware that foods with dairy products, including unpasteurized milk, ice cream, mayonnaise, and egg dishes, can easily be contaminated.

- Be very cautious about open shared dishes, such as salad dressing or salsa and dips put on your table, and open food containers, such as those at salad bars or buffets.

As the newspapers regularly attest, you do not have to leave the country to experience the dangers of hazardous food. If you have taken all the necessary precautions and you still find yourself suffering from intestinal distress, contact a competent medical facility. (Also see "Intestinal Difficulties" later in this chapter.)

If You or Your Children Get Sick Away from Home

Research your options for medical care before you leave home and when you arrive at your destination. If someone in your family becomes ill, you will be especially grateful for all the time you spent preparing for your vacation. Think, too, about bringing a picture or phrase book asking common medical questions in the local language.

Your list of important phone numbers should include medical facilities at your destination. Most large cities have children's hospitals affiliated with a medical school and/or travel clinic. Many American embassies are also knowledgeable about obtaining medical care. Or, check with your credit card or travel insurance company.

If someone does get sick and time permits, first telephone your own physician for advice. If your health emergency is not immediately life threatening, you might want to consider flying home to be treated by your personal physician.

If the problem is life threatening, try to secure ambulance service. Otherwise, in some cities the fastest way to a hospital emergency room may be by taxi or hotel shuttle. Do not be shy about asking your hotel to supply transportation. It is safer to use a taxi service known to the hotel than to rely on independents.

If you are staying in a hotel in the United States or Canada and you need a doctor to come to your hotel room, call (800) HOTEL–DR (468–3537). This San Diego–based company lists 2,500 on-call physicians.

If you are treated abroad, bring back home with you documents about your evaluation and treatment.

If you or your child must go to a hospital, consider the following:

- Does the hospital have twenty-four-hour physician coverage for major trauma, as well as specialists and doctors who speak English?

- Are departments available for intensive care, coronary care, obstetrics, and pediatrics, with appropriate diagnostic equipment, such as ultrasound, CT, and MRI?

- Is the hospital clean, with appropriate lab, blood bank facilities, and disposable syringes?

- What type of payment is accepted?

Infectious Disease and Immunization

As you are planning your travels, allow yourself plenty of time to research current health conditions and obtain necessary immunizations. The risk of infectious diseases is greater in developing countries. Work with your physicians to get a combination of preventive medications that is right for you, for your child, and for your destination. Here are some points to consider in your planning:

- Begin your research four to six months in advance of your travels. Some immunizations require several doses administered over a period of time.

- The Centers for Disease Control and Prevention (CDC) provides current information for travelers by phone, fax, and on-line. Call (877) FYI–TRIP (394–8747), fax (888) 232–3299, or visit its site at www.cdc.gov/travel.

- Pay special attention to the needs of more vulnerable travelers, such as small children, pregnant or lactating women, immunocompromised individuals, and the elderly.

- Be sure you and your child are up to date on routine vaccinations (usually completed in childhood). Some diseases that are largely eradicated in the United States, such as polio, may still pose a threat in other countries, so check your medical records.

- Talk with your doctor, travel clinic, health department, and/or the CDC about recommended vaccinations for your destinations.

- Young children put everything, including their hands, in their mouths. Frequent hand washing is an important disease-control measure for both children and adults. Antibacterial waterless hand-washing lotions are widely available in small, easy-to-carry bottles and offer some protection if soap and water are unavailable.

- Some medications and vaccinations are not available for children under two years of age; check with your pediatrician or a travel medicine clinic.

- Sick children, especially infants with vomiting and/or diarrhea, are at a greater risk of dehydration. Fluid replacement is crucial. Talk with your doctor about oral rehydrating solutions in solution or dry packet form. If a balanced rehydrating solution is not available, a simple fluid replacement solution can be made as follows: To 250 ml (about one mug) of boiled water, add a finger-pinch of salt, one teaspoon of sugar, and a squeeze of orange juice for flavor and potassium. Allow to cool before administering.

- Children traveling in developing countries may be prone to diarrhea. Again, ask your pediatrician about oral rehydrating solutions and about the BRAT diet (Bananas, Rice/rice cereal, Applesauce, and Toast/crackers) to firm stools once liquids are tolerated well.

- Apply insect repellant with care on infants, along with protective clothing.

- Rabies is more common in developing countries. Keep young children away from stray dogs. (See "Animal Concerns, Including Rabies" below.)

- Malaria protection is crucial, especially today, with more resistant strains. When you are traveling, or after you return home, malaria may be the cause of otherwise unexplained fever. (See "Malaria" below.)

- Hepatitis diseases are often confusing. As of this printing, vaccines are available only for Hepatitis A and Hepatitis B, including an A/B combined vaccine (Twinrix) for people eighteen and older. (See "Hepatitis" below.)

- Use common sense when purchasing food. Food purchased from street vendors or at festivals or carnivals may pose additional, unnecessary risk.

- Local baby-sitters may expose your children to infectious diseases.

- If you see a doctor for any reason when you return home, be sure to mention that you have been traveling and where you have been.

Vaccine Considerations

An important part of your planning is learning the disease prevention strategies for your travel destination. Your travel plans may affect or interfere with routine vaccinations—and your need for travel immunization may disrupt your established vaccination timetable. Check with your pediatrician, family physician, travel clinic, and the CDC for updated information on current conditions and recent disease outbreaks.

Travel immunizations are especially important for:

- visitors to high-risk endemic or epidemic regions, especially rural areas

- young children or adults over fifty with health risks; all travelers over sixty-five years of age

- those who have never been vaccinated (for example, adults at risk for chicken pox)

- prolonged stays in areas of high risk or exposure to local people

- international travelers working the health care facilities

- travelers who do not have a spleen or are immunocompromised

Be prepared for your pretravel doctor's appointment with the following information:

- age; past medical history, including routine and travel vaccinations; travel history; and current health status for each adult and child traveling

- all intended destinations, both familiar and remote, and duration of travel

- type of lodging and eating facilities to be used

- anticipated contact with local people through work, baby-sitters, markets, and so forth

- if you are pregnant or lactating

Make certain that your children's standard immunizations are up-to-date. Routine immunizations in the United States for children up to five years of age are usually as follows:

- chicken pox (varicella)—one shot

- diphtheria, tetanus, and pertussis (DTaP)—usually five shots

- haemophilus influenza type b (Hib)—three or four shots

- hepatitis A (HAV)—currently optional for school, one shot and a booster six to twelve months or eighteen months later (depending on vaccine)

- hepatitis B (HBV)—three shots

- measles, mumps, and rubella (MMR)—two shots

- pneumococcal conjugate vaccine (Prevnar)—three or four shots (depending on when shots are started, usually two to twenty-four months of age)

- polio (injectable polio vaccine—IPV—only available in the United States)—four shots

Be sure you are current on your routine immunizations as an adult. For example, adults may not be aware that tetanus-diphtheria immunizations should be repeated every ten years. Depending upon your destination, ask your doctor about the advisability of travel vaccines or other treatments for the following:

- chicken pox—Also known as varicella. Immunization is routine for children. It is important for adults and adolescents who are not immunized. Serious complications may occur.

- cholera—A vaccine is available in Canada but not currently available in the United States; confirm requirement for vaccine or medical exemption letter.

- hepatitis A—This is typically contracted from improper food handling by a person with hepatitis A; it is approved in the United States for children two and up, with two shots administered six to eighteen months apart, depending on the vaccine.

- hepatitis B—Three shots are required for children by kindergarten. For adults eighteen and older, the Twinrix vaccine is available for hepatitis A and B in two shots.

- influenza—Travel increases exposure to this viral disease; in the United States, a vaccine is seasonally available to individuals over fifty and to those with respiratory ailments and compromised immune conditions.

- Japanese encephalitis (JE—Three shots are approved for ages one and up. JE is spread between farm animals and people by mosquitoes; common in rice paddies and pig farms.

- malaria—No vaccines are available; prophylactic medication before, during, and after travel; check with the CDC or a travel physician for current medications; additional information follows below.

- measles, mumps, and rubella—Some adults may need a booster. Two shots are required for children by kindergarten.

- meningococcal meningitis—This is especially important for young adults entering college and in the military, as well as travelers going to epidemic regions.

- polio—Check each individual's immunization record; a booster may be required. Four or five shots are required for children by kindergarten.

- rabies—This is especially important in developing countries for children who are friendly with animals.

- tetanus/diphtheria—A childhood series of five shots is required by kindergarten. A booster every ten years after the initial childhood series is required. Many adults are not properly immunized.

- tuberculosis—A PPD skin test before and after travel may be important, especially if traveling to high-risk areas. Check with your doctor.

- typhoid—This bacterial disease comes from contaminated food and water; a vaccine is available only in the United States.

- yellow fever—Certification of immunization may be required for entry into specific countries. The vaccine is not administered to infants younger than four months. Outbreaks have increased in the last several years.

A physician who specializes in travel medicine may be particularly helpful if you are traveling to developing countries or if you or members of your family have chronic medical conditions. Having the most current information on vaccines and disease outbreaks not only can protect your family's health, but it can provide you with peace of mind and make your trip more enjoyable.

Some Diseases to Be Aware Of

Amebiasis

Amebiasis is a serious parasitic infection of the large intestine that can move into the liver. It is transmitted by eating food contaminated with fecal matter or through person-to-person contact, including sexual contact. The parasite is commonly found in Mexico, South America, and Africa. The condition may progress from a mild state, with few or no symptoms, to amebic dysentery, accompanied by fever and extreme abdominal distress. It is treated with antibiotics.

Cholera

Cholera is an acute intestinal infection. It occurs in many of the developing countries of Africa and Asia where sanitary conditions are poor. Cholera outbreaks have also occurred recently in parts of Latin America.

The organism that causes the illness is spread by ingestion of food or water contaminated directly or indirectly by infected persons. The best protection is to avoid consuming food or water that may be contaminated. The organism can grow well in some foods, such as rice, but will not grow or survive in very acidic foods, including carbonated beverages. It is killed by heat.

Most infected persons have no symptoms or only mild diarrhea. However, persons who are severely affected by the disease can die within a few hours after onset due to loss of fluid and salts through profuse diarrhea and, to a lesser extent, through vomiting.

Where there is the possibility of cholera, see a physician immediately. Do not risk waiting forty-eight hours to see if a severe case of diarrhea will cease.

Treatment for cholera involves rehydration with oral rehydration solutions or, in the most severe cases, with intravenous solutions until the patient is able to ingest fluids. Treatment with antibiotics (usually tetracycline or doxycycline) may decrease the duration of illness and the volume of fluid lost.

The only licensed cholera vaccine in the United States has been discontinued because it offered only brief and incomplete immunity. Recently developed vaccines for cholera are licensed and available in other countries. Check with the CDC for the most current updates.

Giardiasis

Giardiasis is a parasitic disease caused by exposure to food and water contaminated with human or animal fecal matter. The parasites are also found in mountain streams and ponds, giving the name "backpacker's diarrhea" to the condition. It can be transmitted among individuals through close personal contact and poor hygiene, especially lack of hand washing.

The parasite may cause a variety of intestinal symptoms. However, if you have worsening diarrhea, you should see a physician. Giardiasis is treated with antibiotics. Hand washing, safe food handling, and use of safe water are valuable prevention measures.

Hepatitis

Hepatitis A through E (and F and G more recently reported) are serious viral diseases that can affect the liver, causing acute and chronic morbidity and mortality, which should be of concern to everyone. (Other agents and toxins that can cause hepatitis are beyond the scope of this book.) Parents as well as doctors should be aware of the vaccinations available for hepatitis A and B. In Canada infants can be immunized against hepatitis A when they are over one year of age; in the United

States they must be over two years of age. Other countries may vary, so discuss this with your physician.

In the United States, most children are required to be immunized against hepatitis B with a three-shot series by age five or six (before kindergarten). Many parents think that this immunization includes hepatitis A, but it does not.

A more recent vaccine that protects against hepatitis A and B, Twinrix, is available for those over eighteen years of age. It is a three-shot series over a six-month period, replacing the five shots required individually for hepatitis A and B. The chart on the next page provides a brief overview of the various types of viral hepatitis. More detailed descriptions follow.

Common symptoms, such as fatigue, fever, decreased appetite, jaundice (yellow skin), dark urine, and abdominal pain may or may not be present with viral hepatitis. Being proactive, careful, and aware of the seriousness of the hepatitis group is crucial for all travelers.

A brief discussion of hepatitis A through E follows to provide additional details and reduce confusion regarding this escalating problem.

Hepatitis A is the "food handling" type of hepatitis previously called infectious hepatitis. It is transmitted person to person via fecal or oral contamination. You can get hepatitis A anywhere people handle and serve food. The acute disease is usually milder than hepatitis B but can progress to a severe condition. Two hepatitis A vaccines are currently licensed in the United States; neither is approved for children under two years old. Two shots are required, the second one six, twelve, or eighteen months after the first, depending on the vaccine. This provides immunity for those over seven years of age. (See "Hepatitis B" below for information about the combined vaccine, Twinrix.)

Hepatitis B is a highly acute and chronic contagious disease transmitted via body fluids or blood that is infected. Carriers may have asymptomatic chronic hepatitis that progresses to complications and liver failure. Vaccines are available only for hepatitis A and B at the moment. Most children are immunized (three shots) by the time they are five years of age. A new combined vaccine, called Twinrix, is available for hepatitis A and B. Everyone eighteen years of age and older should be immunized against hepatitis A and B!

Hepatitis C, a blood-borne virus, is sometimes called the silent epidemic. The CDC estimates that more than 2.7 million people are chronically infected and may have the disease for ten to twenty years before symptoms appear. More than three-quarters of the people who get the disease become chronic carriers. Much research is being done to improve treatment regimens, but no vaccine is currently available. At the moment, interferon and ribavirin are being given together for

VIRAL HEPATITIS A – E

	Hepatitis A (HAV)	Hepatitis B (HBV)	Hepatitis C (HCV)	Hepatitis D (HDV)	Hepatitis E (HEV)
Means of transmission	food, water, enteric, blood (rare)	blood bodily fluids	blood	blood	food, water, enteric
Most common risk factors	food, water contamination anal-to-hand contact, exposure where children gather	IV drug abuse, sexual contact (especially multiple), occupational exposure	IV drugs, transfusions before 1992, occupational exposure, long-term dialysis	IV drugs, sexual contact, presence of hepatitis B virus	endemic in undeveloped countries
Incubation period	4 weeks average, 15–50 days	50 days average, 1 to 6 months	6 to 7 weeks average, 2 to 26 weeks	2 to 8 weeks	2 to 9 weeks
Clinical course	more acute, usually less chronic	very infectious; acute leading to chronic	most chronic viral infection in the U.S. "Silent epidemic"	acute and chronic	complications especially in pregnant women
Immunization available	HAV vaccine (2 shots) or Twinrix (hepatitis A & B) if over 18 years of age	HBV vaccine (3 shots) or Twinrix (hepatitis A & B) if over 18 years of age	none	HBV vaccine protects against HDV	none
Postexposure treatment	Possible with immuno-globulin	Possible with immuno-globulin	none	none	none

treatment. Because of the elevated risk of hepatitis C, it is highly desirable to avoid medical treatment that might require shots or blood transfusion while in developing countries.

Hepatitis D can only be active when hepatitis B is also present. The viral hepatitis, transmitted by body fluids and blood, is found mostly in chronic HBV carriers, especially in South America and around the Mediterranean.

Hepatitis E, like hepatitis A, is usually transmitted by fecal or oral contact through improper food handling. Diligent attention to food and water can reduce the possibility of hepatitis E as well as A. It is most prevalent in tropical and sub-tropical countries, where it typically affects young adults. There is a particular risk to pregnant women and their unborn children. There is currently no vaccine or other treatment available, and all caution should be taken to achieve sanitary conditions for food and water. Trials for a vaccine are now in progress.

Hepatitis F (French) virus seems close to HAV and HEV in how it is transmitted.

Hepatitis G is related to HCV. It is found in over 30 percent of children who have had transfusions.

Hepatitis F and G are being studied extensively to develop testing and treatments.

Lyme Disease

Lyme disease results from infection by spirochetes transmitted to humans by the bite of infected deer ticks present in certain locations in the northeast, north central, and Pacific coastal regions of North America and in temperate forested areas of Europe and Asia. If possible, avoid tick habitats in areas with a history of Lyme disease. If exposure cannot be avoided, apply repellents to skin and pesticides that kill mites and ticks to clothing. Also make daily checks for any attached ticks. Symptoms of Lyme disease include a rash at the site of the tick bite, fatigue, aches and pains, headache, fever, and chills. There was a vaccine for Lyme disease in the United States, but it has been discontinued. Early intervention with antibiotics is usually effective.

Malaria

One of the greatest hazards of exotic travel is also one of the smallest: the mosquito. The mosquito bite sustained in your backyard may be itchy and annoying, but the bite you get on an international vacation could be deadly.

As Americans have ventured further and further afield in search of new travel experiences, they have encountered mosquito-borne malaria in ever-greater numbers. There are four types of malarial parasites, which are carried by mosquitoes and transferred to the human bloodstream by the mosquito's bite. Although the disease (but not the pest!) was generally eliminated within the United States in the 1940s, it continues to be a deadly threat in more than one hundred other countries. According to the Centers for Disease Control (CDC), 300 to 500 million cases of malaria are diagnosed (90 percent of them in Africa) and some two million deaths—half of them children under five—result from the disease each year.

Of the 1,200 cases of malaria diagnosed annually in the United States, most are among those populations who have spent time in countries where the disease is endemic—travelers and immigrants. Typically, a couple of weeks after returning from their vacation, travelers will start to experience flu-like symptoms. Treated quickly by a knowledgeable physician, the disease can be managed. However, if the symptoms are ignored or if the person is treated by a doctor unfamiliar with the disease, the results can be devastating. (The CDC indicates that most people begin to experience symptoms ten days to four weeks after the bite, but symptoms may appear as quickly as eight days or be delayed as long as a year.)

In most cases malaria is a preventable disease. The CDC recommends that travelers to known malarial countries follow these steps:

- Consult a physician four to six weeks prior to travel. Look for a physician who is knowledgeable about hazards to travelers and specifically about malaria. Be sure you understand dosage and timing and ask about side effects of antimalarial medication.

- Consider postponing travel to malarial countries if you are expecting. Not all antimalarial medications are suitable for pregnant women.

- Be aware that prescriptions for children are based on the child's weight, and doses must be given very carefully. Many of the medications are bitter and can be specially prepared by a pharmacist in a form that will mix with sweetened foods. Fortunately Malarone, a new antimalarial with a pediatric formulation liquid, is now available.

- Take prescribed medications exactly as instructed. Generally you will begin the medication prior to leaving home and continue taking it during travel and for some time after you return, as directed.

- Use insect repellents with DEET and follow your doctor's instructions carefully. The American Academy of Pediatrics recommends 10 percent DEET for children; in high-risk areas, some physicians raise that to 30 percent.

- Wear protective clothing, especially long pants and long-sleeved shirts, and be particularly vigilant in the evening hours when mosquitoes are busiest.

- Sleep under a bed net that has been treated with insecticide.

- Know the symptoms of malaria and see a doctor immediately if you or your child begins to experience any symptoms, such as fever, fatigue, or headache.

Chloroquine used to be a nearly universal preventive medication, but today it is useless in many regions of the world where the rapidly mutating parasite has become resistant to its effects. Be sure to discuss your itinerary with your doctor. If you are traveling to different regions of the world, the same antimalarial medication may not be effective in all areas. Depending on your destination, your physician may prescribe Aralen (chloroquine), doxycycline, Malarone, or Plaquenil (hydroxy-chloroquine sulfate). Treatments vary significantly in cost—and in side effects. Side effects may be significant, so they should be discussed carefully with your physician. But the disease, which can relapse even after treatment, is certainly worse.

The CDC advises: "Any traveler who becomes ill with a fever or flu-like illness while traveling and up to one year after returning home should immediately seek professional medical care. You should tell your health care provider that you have been traveling in a malaria-risk area."

For more complete information visit the Centers for Disease Control Web site at www.cdc.gov/travel.

Salmonella

Salmonella enteritis is an intestinal illness typically caused by contact with an infected animal, such as in food preparation, or by eating undercooked, contaminated food. Salmonella bacteria are commonly found in poultry, livestock, rodents, and reptiles, and it is not unusual for household pets to be infected. If the bacteria enter the bloodstream, the condition can be life threatening.

There is no vaccine for salmonella enteritis, but by following the safe food and water instructions found at the beginning of this chapter, most problems can be avoided. If fever and intestinal problems arise, see a doctor. The condition is treated effectively with antibiotics.

Schistosomiasis

This disease, also known as bilharzia, is caused by parasitic worms called schistosomes. The infection occurs when skin comes in contact with contaminated freshwater in which certain types of snails that carry schistosomes are living. Freshwater can be contaminated by schistosome eggs when infected people urinate or defecate in the water. Schistosomes can penetrate the skin of persons who are wading, swimming, bathing, or washing in contaminated water. Within several weeks, worms grow inside the blood vessels of the body and produce eggs. Some of these eggs travel to the bladder or intestines and are passed into the urine or stool.

If you live in or travel to areas where schistosomiasis occurs and your skin comes in contact with freshwater from canals, rivers, streams, or lakes, you are at risk of getting schistosomiasis. Avoid swimming or wading in freshwater, although swimming in the ocean and in chlorinated swimming pools is generally safe. Be especially careful to drink only safe water. You must assume that all water coming directly from canals, lakes, rivers, streams, or springs is unsafe.

Shigellosis

Also known as *bacillary dysentery,* shigellosis is easily transmitted between people through contact with contaminated food or by flies, which carry the bacteria. Symptoms include rapid-onset fever, cramps, diarrhea—often bloody—and other abdominal distress. It is treated with antibiotics.

Typhoid Fever

Typhoid fever is a bacterial disease contracted by consuming contaminated food or water or through contact with an infected person. Symptoms may include flu-like fever and chills, diarrhea, aches and pains, and a rash on the abdomen and chest. There are a number of resistant strains of the bacteria, but if treatment is started immediately, it is usually effective. Be especially vigilant about sanitation; eat only fruits you can peel yourself, avoid salads and iced drinks, and drink only bottled beverages. There is a typhoid vaccine available in the United States; consult with your physician about whether it is advisable for your travels.

Yellow Fever

Yellow fever is a viral disease transmitted between humans by a mosquito. It occurs in certain jungle locations of South America and Africa. General precautions to avoid mosquito bites should be followed. These include the use of insect repellent, protective clothing, and mosquito netting. Yellow fever can cause significant illness in travelers, and most countries have regulations and requirements for yellow fever vaccination that must be met prior to entering the country.

Yellow fever vaccine may be required for entry into certain countries of Africa and South America. After immunization, an International Certificate of Vaccination is issued and will meet entry requirements for all persons traveling to or arriving from countries where there is active or the potential for yellow fever transmission. The certificate is good for ten years. Most countries will accept a medical waiver for persons with a medical contraindication to vaccination (for example, infants younger than four months old, pregnant women, persons hypersensitive to eggs, or those with an immunosuppressed condition).

Important: If anyone in your party will need a medical waiver, obtain it in writing from consular or embassy officials before departure.

Contact state or local health departments for the most recent recommendations or check the CDC Web site: www.cdc.gov/travel. Consult your local health department for yellow fever vaccination sites near you.

The information above introduces some of the more dangerous infectious diseases that affect travelers. Although there are other potentially serious diseases that are not included here, there are many excellent reference books that offer detailed discussion and helpful information. See Appendix C for additional resource information.

Common Travel Problems

This section will help you with many common health problems that may arise as you travel. Whether traveling in the United States or in another country, taking children along presents unique challenges in preventing and managing illnesses and accidents. Because children and adolescents will usually be traveling with their parents and the family will have similar injury and risk exposures, general information about managing typical illnesses in family members is presented, with a special emphasis on children.

Your physician will be able to advise you if you or your child have chronic or recurring problems that may affect your plans. In addition renewing your first-aid and CPR certification prior to your trip will prepare you to handle the unexpected.

Allergies

Allergies is a term that covers a wide spectrum of conditions from hay fever, allergic rhinitis, and eczema to asthma (usually a more chronic condition) and allergic reactions to bee stings.

If you or your children have allergies, take a large supply of regular medications in their original containers. If you are flying, keep allergy medications in your carry-on luggage. If you have allergic reactions, especially to medications (such as penicillin), foods, or stinging insects (bees, wasps, and hornets), ask your physician about what you should do in the event of a severe reaction. In such a case, an epinephrine injection may be a lifesaver. (Epi-Pen, premeasured auto injections, require a prescription.) If you or your children are allergic to particular plants, pollens, molds, or animals, ask your physician or allergist about potential exposures before your trip.

Anaphylaxis

Anaphylaxis is a severe allergic reaction that can result in major illness or death. For some people the allergic reaction after exposure is immediate; for others it may not occur until the second or third exposure. It is therefore difficult to determine how someone might react to a future exposure.

Possible allergens can include chemicals, a variety of foods and food additives, insect stings, drugs, vaccines, latex, or even strenuous exercise. The symptoms that are most commonly associated with anaphylaxis include itchiness or hives; swelling of the throat, face, and tongue; difficulty breathing; vomiting; light-headedness; falling blood pressure; and shock; to name a few.

After an individual is exposed, symptoms can occur within one to fifteen minutes of contact. Emergency care should begin immediately, including using an Epi-Pen, calling 911 or other knowledgeable help, and ambulance transportation to the nearest emergency room.

If you or your child has a severe allergy, talk with your pediatrician and carry epinephrine kits at home, school or work, and in your travel medicine kit.

Animal Concerns, Including Rabies

Since rabies is well managed among domestic animals in the United States, few travelers consider the risk of this viral disease. But in many parts of the world, including most of Central and South America, India, Asia, and Africa, rabies is common enough to account for some 40,000 deaths each year.

Rabies is transmitted through the bite of a rabid animal. Carried in the animal's saliva, it attacks the nervous system of humans and is almost always fatal if untreated. Although it is carried by cats, cattle, coyotes, bats, skunks, raccoons, and foxes, according to the CDC, "exposure to rabid dogs is still the cause of over 90 percent of human exposures to rabies and of over 99 percent of human deaths worldwide." Afflicted animals can be deadly without showing noticeable symptoms.

This hazard makes it especially important to teach small children appropriate behavior around unfamiliar animals. A small child's friendly pat can easily be rewarded with a bite to the hand or face.

In case of animal bite, wash the area with soap and water, apply an antiseptic, and get medical help immediately at a hospital emergency room.

If you are traveling outside the United States, and especially if you will be visiting developing countries, talk with your physician about the advisability of pre-exposure vaccinations. They are less costly and less traumatic than post-bite vaccinations, which must be initiated immediately and which may be advised if there is any possibility that the animal is rabid. Contact the U.S. embassy for additional help.

The Centers for Disease Control has extensive information on rabies on its Web site at www.cdc.gov, or by phone at (800) 311–3435.

An animal safety consideration is the petting zoo or farm visit. Petting zoos have become popular at fairs, carnivals, farms, and special events for children and warrant a wise parent's attention.

Although petting zoo animals are selected for their mild demeanor, they can still bite if provoked. But the greater concern is for exposure to bacterial infections, including e. coli and salmonella. In the petting area, avoid hand-mouth activities, such as eating and drinking, or carrying items, such as pacifiers, that might end up in a child's mouth. Be especially watchful of toddlers. Never touch an animal that appears sick. Wash hands thoroughly with soap and water after touching animals or spending time in animal enclosures.

The U.S. Department of Agriculture sets standards and certifies petting zoos for proper animal care and conditions. A certified petting zoo is less likely to present a hazard to visitors.

Back Problems

If you or your child has back pain, discuss this with your doctor before your trip. Consider using a hot-water bottle or heating pad to relieve pain and muscle spasm. To avoid burns, do not sleep on a heating pad, and be particularly careful about using heating pads to treat back pain in young children. Some tips to help you avoid back pain include the following:

- On long flights or when riding in a vehicle for a long period, place a pillow in the small of your back—preferably a porous one that allows air to circulate.

- If possible, stand up and walk around every forty-five to sixty minutes. If it is not safe or practical to stand, raise and lower your heels and stretch your legs as you remain seated.

- Tall adults and adolescents should try to get a bulkhead or an aisle seat so they can stretch their legs. Adults and children whose feet do not reach the floor may benefit from putting something on the floor to act as a footrest.

- When driving a vehicle, adjust the seat so that your knees are at about a thirty-degree angle above your hips when your feet are touching the pedals. Stop approximately once an hour to walk around and stretch.

- Avoid the extra soft chairs and couches that are common in hotel rooms and lobbies; soft furniture places abnormal strain on the back.

- Kneeling on a chair when bending over a bathroom sink to wash your hair prevents undue stress on the lower back.

- To lift heavy objects, stand close to the object, squat down, keep your back straight, and lift mostly with your legs rather than with your arms.

- Avoid walking around in ski boots and wearing shoes with heels more than 1½ inches high.

- A regular walking or swimming program usually helps alleviate back problems and, if possible, should be continued during a vacation. Although regular exercise is often the best treatment for recurrent back pain, a vacation is not a good time to start such a program. If you or your child plan to participate in a sporting vacation, get in shape for the sport before you travel, even if it means postponing the trip for another year.

- Acute back pain can be helped with pain medications, hot baths or showers for spasms, ice applications, and sleeping on a firm surface such as a firm mattress, bed boards, or mattress without springs on the floor. Heating pads and ice bags that are portable and chemically activated by adding water are commonly available in pharmacies and travel stores.

- Bed rest helps back pain in the short term; however, in the long term, people who stay active and tolerate a reasonable amount of pain have less back pain than those who overdo bed rest. When bed rest seems helpful, lie first on one side and then on the other while curled up, or on your back with a support under your knees. Do not lie on your stomach.

Bites—Animal and Human

Bites are most common among children between kindergarten and fifteen years of age, especially in the summer. About a million and a half animal bites are reported each year, with emergency room visits common for secondary infections. Dog bites account for about a quarter of all bites, but cat bites develop more secondary infections. Puncture wounds are harder to clean and have a high incidence of secondary infection because bacteria are forced deep into the tissue.

Along with extensive wound cleaning and aggressive treatment of infected bites, a thorough history and physical examination of the patient and the animal is important. In taking the animal's history, ask:

1. Was the animal wild or domestic?

2. Did the animal seem sick or healthy?

3. Do you know the status of the animal's rabies immunization?

4. How did it happen? Was the bite provoked?

5. Is rabies known to be prevalent in this location?

In taking the patient's history, the following questions are important:

1. Is the patient up to date on immunizations?

2. Are there any known present illnesses?

3. Are there any medication allergies?

4. In an area where rabies is present, especially rural areas, did the patient have immunization against rabies?

Human bites are potentially more serious than cat and dog bites and require aggressive washing and proper medical treatment. Do not use steristrips, tight bandages, or sutures, which may enclose an infection.

In the case of an animal or human bite, wash the area thoroughly with soap and water. Watch carefully for redness and swelling at the site, especially during the first three days after the bite. Consult a physician; proper treatment with antibiotics is crucial to good healing.

Animal, especially dog, bites are more common when an animal is provoked. Be proactive in educating your children about animal safety.

Burns

Burns can happen at any age. Common causes of burns are curling irons, flat irons, barbecue coals and grills, sparklers and fireworks, and, of course, hot spilled items and stove mishaps.

A first-degree burn causes redness. A second-degree burn causes blistering. In either case, cool the burned area as soon as possible by immersing it in water. Ice is no longer recommended. Clean the area carefully with soap and water or cotton swabs and a dilute solution of hydrogen peroxide. To prevent infection, apply bacterial cream and a nonstick dressing, especially if the burn is blistered and painful. More severe burns, especially deeper or possibly third-degree burns, must be given medical treatment immediately.

Choking

Choking is frightening and can be fatal at any age, but it is especially dangerous for children five and under when air passages are small and curiosity is large. Any small object—food, toy, bean, marble, coin, button, balloon, cigarette butt, pill, twig—can be stuffed into mouth, nose, or ear in an unsupervised moment. Even the most common foods, such as nuts, hot dogs, raw vegetables, fruits, hard candy, popcorn, and others, can block the airway.

Classes on child and infant first aid and CPR (cardiopulmonary resuscitation) cover the subject of choking in detail and are highly recommended, especially before you take a trip.

If a person who is choking is coughing, he or she may be able to dislodge the object. If the person is gagging or cannot breathe, he or she is choking and in need of immediate assistance. Call 911 (in the United States) or the best medical help available. Adults and children as young as twelve months who are choking but conscious can be given the Heimlich maneuver, which can help the victim to dislodge something that is blocking the airway. The Heimlich maneuver is covered in CPR classes. Never slap or pound a person on the back if they are coughing or choking. This may lodge the object deeper in the airway.

If the person collapses, you will need to attempt rescue breathing and continue trying to dislodge the object. As long as the person has a pulse, you can alternate between rescue breathing attempts and the Heimlich maneuver, checking regularly for resumed breathing and pulse. If the heart stops, you must begin CPR, while still attempting to dislodge the object.

Even if you succeed in dislodging the object and restoring the person to consciousness, the victim should always see a physician after a serious choking incident.

Constipation

See "Intestinal Difficulties."

Cuts and Abrasions

Cuts and abrasions are one of the most common reasons parents take their children to doctors' offices and emergency rooms. It may be difficult to stay calm when your child is bleeding, but a calm assessment is essential to proper care.

Use direct pressure on cuts for at least five minutes. Remember that some body parts, such as the scalp and the chin, are more vascular and will bleed profusely. If after ten minutes bleeding has not stopped, the child should be seen by a doctor. Many cuts can now be "glued" together, thus avoiding stitches completely. If the cut is gaping or has ragged edges, especially on the face or lip borders, a doctor should be consulted to evaluate and possibly suture the wound.

Wash cuts and abrasions well with soap and water and remove foreign material, such as dirt and broken glass, if you can get it out easily. If not, seek medical help. Apply an antibacterial ointment or cream and bandage with nonstick gauze.

Signs of infection, such as redness and swelling, usually appear one to five days after the injury.

A secondary bacterial skin infection, *impetigo,* may form in a break in the skin as "honey-crusted" lesions surrounded with redness. Good cleaning, removal of the crusts with peroxide, local antibiotics (Bactroban, by prescription), and oral antibiotics, at times, are necessary. Another superficial secondary skin infection around hair follicles, *folliculitis,* can usually be treated in much the same way.

Dental Issues

Take floss and extra toothbrushes with you on any trip. A dental checkup before your trip will help you and your child avoid a toothache or other dental problems while traveling. If a filling, cap, or crown gets loose or broken while you are traveling, covering the area with dental wax or gum may help reduce pain. Preparations for this purpose can be bought in most pharmacies and travel stores and are a sensible item to add to your travel first-aid kit.

If possible, avoid going to an unknown dentist. In some countries, dentists pull teeth that in the United States would be repaired. Avoid having a tooth pulled until you return home and can see your own dentist.

If you must see a dentist while traveling, go to one whose office is clean, whose instruments have been properly sanitized, and who uses needles only one time before discarding them.

Diarrhea

See "Intestinal Difficulties."

Ear Problems

Children who have a cold or have had recurrent ear infections are a particular challenge. Ear infection or persistent ear pain associated with altitude changes, such as mountain driving or airplane travel, can be difficult to manage away from home. If you think your child is at risk of an earache, see your physician before traveling. You may want to postpone the trip until your child gets over the cold.

If your ears ache when you fly or feel stuffed up, you are not alone. Most people have no significant ear problems, but many people suffer from *airplane ears*. The causes for this are simple. As an airliner descends to land, cabin air pressure increases, causing the eardrum to retract slightly. This prevents the eustachian tubes (between nose and mouth) from opening and allowing the pressure to equalize. The unequal pressure on the eardrum causes the clogged feeling, which sometimes leads to temporary hearing loss and even to acute pain. You can ease the distress of airplane ears by following these suggestions:

- If your children have recurrent ear infections and you are traveling in an airplane, have them yawn, chew, and swallow during descent. Be prepared by having gum, food, or drink available at the end of the flight. If your child develops an earache, ask the flight attendant for a warm towel to put over the affected ear.

- Do not wait until your ears hurt to start warding off the problem. As soon as the aircraft begins its descent, swallow or yawn several times. This helps to keep the eustachian tubes open. Hearing slight clicking sounds or a change in the noise level means the pressure is equalizing. For some people, chewing gum or wiggling their lower jaw helps.

- If swallowing, yawning, chewing gum, or wiggling your jaw does not help, gently blow your nose. You can also try this procedure: Hold your nostrils closed with thumb and forefinger, breathe in through your mouth, and then very gently try to breathe out through your nose.

- If you usually experience airplane ears when you fly, stay awake when coming in for a landing. If you are awake you will have more control and a better chance of easing the pressure on your eardrums.

- Avoid alcoholic beverages during your flight. Alcohol causes the mucous membranes and eustachian tubes to swell, making the problem worse.

- Since colds and allergies make this condition worse, try to avoid flying when you are congested. If you must fly, take an over-the-counter or prescription cold tablet an hour before landing. Some who experience chronic ear pain when flying get relief from decongestants, even when they do not have a cold.

- Pressure-regulating earplugs, called EarPlanes, are available without prescription and fit adults and children ages one to eleven years. When used as directed—placed gently in the ears—they may help to equalize ear pressure and reduce the discomfort many people experience during air travel. Avoid using earplugs when severe sinus congestion has completely blocked the eustachian tubes; better to avoid air travel altogether and seek medical help.

Otitis Media (Middle Ear Infection) Otitis media, which occurs when the eardrum or translucent membrane becomes inflamed, is one of the most common illnesses seen in children. It can be acute or chronic. It usually follows a cold or other respiratory condition. Antibiotics may or may not be indicated. Analgesics (see otitis extrema) may be helpful to reduce ear pain. Consult a physician if you or your child has a current problem, and discuss past history of infections with your doctor before leaving on a trip.

Otitis Extrema (Swimmer's Ear) Swimmer's ear, a common inflammation in the ear canal, is most prevalent during the summer months. The ear canal in front of the eardrum can become inflamed and infected when bacteria get beneath the surface of the skin, especially during significant water exposure. The external ear can get quite painful, especially when touched, pulled, or moved. Analgesic ear drops are soothing. Topical antibiotics, used for seven to ten days as directed by a physician, usually treat the condition effectively. Ear drops should be dripped slowly alongside the ear canal for better filling and less blocking.

Warm compresses and/or warm mineral oil in the ear canal may also help to reduce ear pain. Cotton will help keep the drops in place. Elevate the child's head with an extra pillow or hold the child or infant in an upright position.

To help prevent swimmer's ear, commercial products such as Swim Ear may be useful, or you can mix your own solution of half white vinegar (acetic acid) and half rubbing alcohol (some prefer half white vinegar and half hydrogen peroxide), putting four or five drops in each ear after swimming.

With either otitis media or otitis extrema, the combination of analgesic eardrops and Benadryl, or your favorite antihistamine, usually helps to decrease ear pain. Benadryl usually makes children sleepy; always try medications before you travel to make sure they do not have the opposite of the intended effect.

Eye Concerns

Adults use sunglasses to protect their eyes from annoying light rays and wind-borne irritants, but they may forget that children's eyes also need protection. It seems ever more certain that the sun's damage is cumulative, on both skin and eyes. Early protection may have lifelong benefits. Be sure to carry extra glasses, contact lenses, and sunglasses on your trip, as well as a copy of your lens prescription.

The air in airplanes is very dry and can cause *dry eye syndrome.* If your or your child's eyes dry easily, use an artificial-tear solution, which is available in most pharmacies. If eyes become itchy from dust or allergies, ask your physician about taking appropriate decongestant eyedrops such as Naphconr or Visine on your trip.

If any members of your travel group are likely to be involved in sports or other strenuous activities that may cause eye injury, take safety glasses on your trip. Swimming goggles that fit well can help protect the eyes from various pollutants.

Conjunctivitis Conjunctivitis is an inflammation of the "whites" of the eyes, which may be bacterial (80 percent), or viral (20 percent), or caused by allergies. Bacterial and viral conjunctivitis are highly contagious and careful hand washing is a must, both when children touch or rub their eyes and when parents administer eyedrops.

In bacterial conjunctivitis, a discharge may develop in the eyelids or lashes, accompanied by redness. The infection usually lasts for about ten days; a viral infection may last longer, around two weeks.

Warm "soaks" with a washcloth or cotton balls applied gently to the eyelids can be useful. For a simple bacterial infection, antibiotic drops or ointment is commonly prescribed for seven to ten days.

Red, itchy eyes may be caused by exposure to an environmental irritant, including allergies, and may need to be treated.

If you or your child are prone to recurrent conjunctivitis, discuss this problem with your doctor before traveling.

Contact Lenses Pay particular attention if you or your children wear contact lenses. Wearing them too long can cause pain and even blisters on the surface of the eye. Carry extra cleaning and wetting solutions when traveling, and never use saliva as a wetting solution because the bacteria in saliva can damage the cornea. If you are going to an area with little access to medical facilities, ask your physician whether you should take an antibacterial eye ointment with you.

Here are some additional recommendations for contact lens wearers:

- If you just started wearing contact lenses, do not wear them on long trips.

- Avoid wearing contact lenses on long flights, and do not wear them when you sleep, unless approved by your physician.

- Carry ample wetting agents and apply them frequently while in flight or in other low-humidity places, such as hot or dry climates and air-conditioned areas.

- Avoid wearing contact lenses while swimming. Never wear them in hot tubs, because hot tubs frequently contain bacteria than can cause serious eye infections and itchy skin rashes.

- If possible, use only bottled sterile water (not tap water) to clean the lenses.

- Wash your hands thoroughly with soap and water before handling contact lenses to avoid contamination from bacteria or irritants.

Fear of Flying

Whether your fear of flying is recent or long held or inspired by a near-miss experience, terrifying news coverage, or unknown causes, the condition is widely shared, equally paralyzing—and equally treatable.

Fear may be amplified by a feeling of lack of control: An individual who is nervous and jumpy as a car passenger may be perfectly calm and competent behind the wheel. Fear of flying may combine this "out of control" sensation with other common fears, such as a fear of heights, fear of dying, and fear of enclosed spaces.

From the low buzz of anxiety to full-blown terror, fear of flying, or *aerophobia,* is manifest in a wide-ranging set of symptoms that vary from person to person and even, for some individuals, from flight to flight. A normally calm passenger may become anxious and a nervous passenger fearful when bad weather, illness, undesirable seating, unusual plane noises, long delays (and resultant missed connections), recent aviation disasters, "dangerous-looking" passengers, or alcohol are added to the mix.

It is of little benefit to speculate whether the fear of flying is rational or irrational: It is real and it interferes with your ability to travel freely and enjoy the experience. It makes much more sense to acknowledge the fear, assure yourself that it is treatable, and begin immediately to deal with it.

There are as many ways to cope with aerophobia as there are symptoms. Some passengers manage their fear with gestures of faith such as carrying a favorite photo, always sitting in the same seat, or only flying on astrologically auspicious days. Others distract themselves with food, books, or work or numb themselves with prescription medications or alcohol. While any method may work temporarily, some, such as drugs and alcohol, only mask symptoms and may in fact compound the underlying problems. There are many well-established ways to reduce the anxiety of aerophobia and many places to seek help.

Among the most common methods are various types of desensitizing exercises that help you recognize and eliminate the triggers to your fear, which may start long before you get on the plane. These include guided imagery, visualization, and relaxation exercises leading to a step-by-step mastery of the entire experience. Such training also typically includes information about flight and the plane itself, how it works, what kind of noises it makes, and how it is outfitted for safety. You will also learn about weather, in-flight turbulence, and how to get information about airline safety.

Children, especially those between about six and twelve years of age, may also experience some fear of airplanes or flying, especially if they have been exposed to recent news reports of air disasters or if they hear a parent talking about being afraid to fly. In addition to the methods that work for adults—increasing knowledge and desensitizing—children may be helped by talking with flight attendants who are trained to assist panicky passengers.

If you are ready to reduce the fear, there are various places to start. There are numerous books and self-help tapes on the subject, and every airline offers tips for passengers. One of the most comprehensive resources is the on-line service AirSafe.com, where, in addition to general information on airlines and flight safety, you will find a page dedicated to resources for the fearful flyer. For additional help or for more persistent or complicated anxieties, many therapists offer group and individual sessions specifically designed for coping with the fear of flying.

Whatever your approach, do not expect instant results and do not be surprised if you have some recurrence of symptoms. Most programs restore and build confidence gradually and benefit from regular "booster" sessions. So, do not wait until the week before your trip. Start today. The sooner you begin, the sooner you will fly with comfort. See Appendix C for recommended books and on-line resources on overcoming or easing the fear of flying.

Foot Matters

Avoid wearing new shoes when traveling. Particularly if your trip is likely to involve a lot of walking or hiking, make sure that your shoes and your child's shoes or boots are well broken-in and comfortable. Wearing thin inner socks and wool outer socks can help protect the feet from friction and blisters. Apply moleskin to sore spots right away to avoid developing blisters. If you have foot problems, seek treatment and advice from a podiatrist before leaving home.

Athlete's foot is common in all kinds of activities, including camping and hiking. Keep your feet as dry as possible. After washing and drying feet, apply an ointment such as Tinactin or Micatin to all areas of the feet, as directed on the package, and continue application for at least a week after the rash is cleared.

Blisters begin with a red tender place on the skin called a *hot spot.* No bubble has yet formed, but if the back and forth rubbing continues, a full-blown blister results. If you catch the hot spot in time, it can be protected with moleskin or molefoam.

Take a piece of moleskin or molefoam three times larger than the hot spot, all around. Fold it in half and cut a hole in the center of the "doughnut" larger than the hot spot. Apply tincture of benzoin around the hot spot or blister to hold the moleskin in place. The hole will help protect the skin. Thicker molefoam may give more protection, depending upon the location of the irritation. Reinforce the moleskin with tape to make it more secure.

If the blister is small, do not puncture it. Let the moleskin protection work. If the blister is large and intact, puncture it and drain the site because the fluid inhibits healing. Trim away the now loose skin and wash the area with soap and water. After dabbing it dry, apply an antibiotic ointment such as Neosporin, Polysporin, or Bactroban (prescription required). Apply a nonadhering sterile dressing or gauze. Use the moleskin protection and check the wound daily. If it gets infected, remove the dressing for drainage and consult a physician right away.

Headache

Headaches are common reasons why children and teenagers see their physicians. Viral infections, allergies, and sinusitis are common causes of acute headaches. Of course, altitude, stress with family or school, and migraines are possible causes as well.

All headaches should be taken seriously in both children and adults. Just as with a stomachache, follow-up evaluations are crucial to determine what associations are related and what makes it better or worse.

Children's Tylenol has an excellent track record for relieving headache. Speak with your doctor and use as little medication as possible because significant side effects can occur.

Head Injury

Head injuries are not uncommon, especially when a child is learning to walk. If the individual loses consciousness, call 911 or seek the best medical help available. If there is no loss of consciousness, closely monitor the person's behavior and call your doctor for medical evaluation or advice, especially if the individual does not act normal for his or her age or shows signs of lethargy, confusion, vomiting, a visible bump, or other abnormal behavior. When in doubt about any of these problems, seek medical help—in person if possible.

High-Altitude Concerns

Many visitors to high altitudes experience distressing symptoms when they first arrive at a new elevation. At a high altitude the body must deal with lower oxygen, lower humidity, and differences in atmospheric pressure. Symptoms can range from mild to severe and may include headache, nausea, and difficulty with breathing.

Here are some hints to ease your adjustment to high altitudes:

- Ascend to higher altitudes gradually. If you are traveling from sea level, stop over at a lower altitude such as 5,000 feet for a day or two before continuing to ascend to higher elevations.

- Increase activity gradually. Sleep late your first morning at a new altitude, then ease into activity—a half day at first, gradually increasing to a full day's activity.

- Eat a light diet. Your diet should be high in carbohydrates and low in fat, with moderate protein. Rich, fatty foods will make you feel worse.

- Increase humidity. As altitude increases, humidity decreases. Your body's reduced moisture may cause increased nasal congestion and thirst. The use of heaters in enclosed areas further reduces moisture. A cold-water vaporizer is good for increasing humidity.

- Increase fluid intake. Drink at least eight ounces every hour: water, fruit juice, or products like Gatorade. Caffeinated or alcoholic beverages aggravate dehydration and should be avoided. If you are so nauseated that you cannot maintain fluid intake, or if the amount you normally urinate decreases, seek medical care immediately. These signs of dehydration can represent a real emergency.

- Be prepared for shortness of breath. Lower air pressure may result in feeling out of breath, especially if you are involved in any kind of physical activity. This should lessen within a few days. If it worsens, or is accompanied by cough, chest pain, or fever, seek immediate medical attention.

- Altitude-related headaches can range from mild to severe. If aspirin, Tylenol for children, or other over-the-counter medications do not help, or if you have signs of confusion, decreased mental sharpness, irritability, or excessive drowsiness, get prompt medical attention. Use common sense; a change in judgment may be the first sign of acute mountain sickness (AMS).

If you live at an elevation that is below 1,000 feet, are over forty, and are neither physically fit nor acclimated to high altitude, you should be wary of engaging in more strenuous physical activity than usual during a quick trip to the mountains. The same applies to overweight children. Even physically fit but unacclimatized children will tire quickly, so be prepared to make them pace themselves during their first days at a high elevation. Tired children are more prone to injury or getting lost.

If you are planning on taking your family hiking in the high country, organize your trip so you can travel to higher altitudes gradually. Aim at gaining no more than 2,000 feet per day over your home's elevation. This will allow everyone's body to adjust to changes in oxygen levels and atmospheric pressures. When possible, do not sleep at the maximum altitude reached each day. Descend to a lower altitude.

Avoid smoking because tobacco smoke compromises your lungs' ability to utilize oxygen. Do not drink alcoholic beverages; they reduce your body's ability to make necessary water and mineral adjustments in your brain.

If you are taking or planning to take any medications, consult your physician about their potential effects at high altitudes. Also, depending on your travel plans, ask your physician whether you should take any medication to help prevent or treat high-altitude problems. (See Appendix C for resources.)

Acute Mountain Sickness Acute mountain sickness can be dangerous. Consider the possibility of acute mountain sickness if you or your child experiences headaches, inability to sleep, dizziness, depression, and/or anxiety after ascending to a high altitude. If altitude sickness is likely, descending about 1,000 feet will usually relieve symptoms. Oxygen, while helpful, is not a cure for altitude sickness. Aspirin or buffered aspirin may help relieve some symptoms for older travelers (check with your doctor).

Homesickness

One of the mysterious maladies of the road is homesickness. It can be intense, especially for children; it can be triggered by a wide variety of events or circumstances; and it can last a few moments or all of the remaining days of your vacation. In its most familiar form, homesickness is a deep nostalgia for the familiar scents, sounds, and sights of home. This is not always bad. The sibling who is a daily rival may turn into a treasured friend from the distance of overnight camp or vacation. On the other hand, persistent homesickness can dampen anyone's enthusiasm for travel. A little preparation goes a long way toward the prevention and reduction of these feelings. Here are some suggestions:

- Before taking an extended trip away from home, "practice" with short outings for a night or two.

- Bring along familiar, comforting items, such as a favorite blanket, toy, or photograph.

- Call a friend at home. Encouraging a homesick child to talk about what he or she has seen and done may give that child a new perspective on time away from home.

- Keep busy. Idle time may allow feelings of homesickness to creep in.

- Set a routine; make it familiar but special. Instead of trying to duplicate home habits while you are on vacation, give your travel routines a special twist. Spend a couple of minutes looking at the stars every night before bed. Start each day with a little present. Turn your child's sleeping area into a "fort." Use your imagination to make places that are new and unfamiliar seem irresistible.

- Encourage your children to participate in the planning for each day's activities. The importance of this role may help them forget that they miss home.

- If you find yourself stuck in a place where the weather is bad, the food is awful, the blankets are scratchy, and there's no immediate way out, a little homesickness is normal. See if you can turn it into something fun. Remember all those movies about the most awful vacations? Make up stories with yourselves as characters, using your current circumstances to set the scene. Keep your sense of humor, and even miserable days can end up being fun!

Hypothermia

Hypothermia occurs when the body loses heat faster than it is produced. Heat loss is commonly caused by exposure to wind and wet clothing, or by immersion in cold water. Excessive perspiration inside wind- and rainproof clothing also increases body-heat loss.

Water-skiers, windsurfers, and participants in other water sports are at risk of hypothermia unless they wear clothing designed to keep them warm. The first noticeable effect of hypothermia from water sports may be persistent chattering teeth. However, hypothermia may cause a drop in the immune system's effectiveness, making the individual more likely to catch a cold or other infection. Severe hypothermia causes a drastic drop in the body's core temperature and can be fatal.

To prevent hypothermia, keep yourself and your child dry and warm. If your trip or activities involve time in or around water or snow, pack towels, extra socks, and dry layers for quick changes.

Injuries and Accidents

Traffic accidents kill far more Americans traveling outside the United States than any other single cause. Accidental injuries from all causes are the most common reasons travelers seek care in emergency rooms, hospitals, and the medical departments of cruise ships. Typical traveler's injuries include ankle sprains, knee injuries, and forearm or wrist fractures. Precautions that may help prevent these injuries include:

- Always wear seatbelts, if available. When traveling with a child younger than four years old, take a car safety seat along, if possible. Injuries are less likely in large vehicles and in rear seats, but seat belts are still essential.

- Take particular care when walking on uneven surfaces, such as cobblestone streets or walkways with potholes, and when stepping off curbs.

- Avoid wearing shoes that have slippery soles, especially on smooth or wet walking surfaces such as cruise ship decks, marbled lobby floors, or wet streets.

- Be particularly careful in and around showers and tubs and other wet surfaces in bathrooms and pool areas.

- Stay alert to your surroundings, even when you are hurrying in a terminal or otherwise distracted by urgent business, to avoid tripping over an object such as a suitcase placed in an inappropriate location.

- Check out each living and play area where your child may spend time. Electrical cords and outlets in many countries do not meet U.S. safety standards. Check barriers, balconies, and furniture for structural integrity.

- When walking at night, use a flashlight if the lighting is inadequate.

- Consider that faucets in foreign countries may be marked differently. For example, "C" may mean hot instead of cold (caliente in Spanish, chaud in French). Because the temperature of hot water sources varies greatly, always test the water first to prevent scalding. This is particularly important when traveling with young children, because they may turn on the hot water faucet and not be able to protect themselves from scalding water.

- Wash cuts and scratches with soap and water as soon as possible and then several times a day to keep them from becoming infected. Two over-the-counter antibiotic ointments, Neosporin and Bacitracin, may be helpful. Bactroban, a very effective topical antibiotic, is available by prescription in the United States.

Insect Bites and Stings

The most common biting insects that cause disease are mosquitoes that bite at dusk or dawn. Travelers may be exposed to insect-transmitted malaria, yellow fever, St. Louis encephalitis, Japanese encephalitis, dengue fever, West Nile virus, and many others. Deer ticks can cause Lyme disease. Additional information on some of these diseases is provided earlier in this chapter in the section "Infectious Disease and Immunization." Check with your travel physician or the CDC regarding hazards in the areas you will be visiting.

Most insect bites are uncomplicated and respond to simple washing. If a stinger is present, remove it with tweezers or scrape it off as quickly as possible. If the area of the bite is very swollen, red, or has radiating red lines, or if the person may be having an allergic reaction, see a physician.

Insect repellent with DEET, applied according to package directions, can prevent bites, as can barrier protection, such as long sleeves, long pants, and netting.

Intestinal Difficulties

The most common digestive irregularities affect people in opposite ways but are alike in this respect: Both tend to knock the enjoyment out of your trip. Here are ways to combat these common distresses.

Abdominal Pain Stomachaches are one of the most common reasons parents bring children or adolescents to their physician. There are a variety of causes, including discomfort from vomiting or diarrhea, family stresses such as a new sibling, and changes of home or school, but, of course, the possibility of appendicitis should be ruled out first. If a child can hop up on a table and down again, or jump up and down at least five times, the chances are small that the discomfort is caused by appendicitis.

Constipation is one of the most common causes of stomachache in children, and many emergency room visits could be avoided if parents would think first about the possibility of constipation.

Constipation Poor diet, not enough fiber, insufficient fluid intake, and not enough exercise all can contribute to this problem, which is also common when a trip involves hurried schedules and dietary changes. Mild constipation is best managed by drinking lots of liquids—more than two or three quarts or liters daily for an older child or adult—and by eating foods that are high in fiber such as bran, whole wheat, fruits, and vegetables.

To relieve constipation, eat the following foods: pitted fruits and their juices, green vegetables, brown rice, bran and whole grain cereals and breads, and snacks such as high fiber bars. Avoid the following: apples, bananas, pears, potatoes, white rice, corn, milk products, white bread, and junk food such as chips and cookies.

Laxative medications that contain fiber include Metamucil, FiberCon, or your favorite one. These medications and 70 percent Sorbitol are safe for long-term use in adolescents and adults. Check with your doctor regarding the use of mineral oil, laxatives, or suppositories.

Stimulant laxatives, such as Dulcolax, are useful for more severe constipation, but they should be used only for a few days. These agents often can also be used by children, but check the labels for age limits and doses. For infants, a barley malt extract such as Maltsupex—one or two teaspoons two or three times daily—is useful.

Diarrhea Diarrhea is one of the most common problems of travelers, especially those under the age of three. It is estimated that over 30 percent of all travelers develop some diarrhea, with the most common causes including diet change and exposure to viruses. The stresses of changing time zones and sleeping patterns can contribute to the intestinal upset.

Discuss with your doctor antimotility medicines, such as Imodium, Pepto Bismol, and others. Many physicians individualize the use of antimotility medications on children and are reluctant to use them on younger children and infants because these medicines slow the entire gut transit of infectious contents and may cause more serious illnesses. Also discuss with a physician knowledgeable in travel medicine the pros and cons of antibiotics, especially if you are going to more rural locations and/or plan a more extended stay in a country with known outbreaks of diseases.

The main risk of diarrhea, especially in young children, is dehydration. Treatment of dehydration requires replacing the body's lost water and minerals. For infants and young children, a balanced solution of water, minerals, and glucose, such as Pedialyte, is safest. Excellent balanced-electrolyte solutions are available today.

In older children or adults, oral rehydrating solutions supplied in packets provide the correct balance of glucose, sodium, potassium, and bicarbonate. For mild diarrhea, a combination of soft drinks—diluted to half strength—and salted soda crackers can be used to replace the lost water and minerals, especially sodium and potassium. High-glucose drinks and foods, such as Gatorade, Jell-O, and nondiet colas, may inhibit absorption.

After initial rehydration, slowly begin to add solid food, such as the well-known BRAT diet (Bananas, Rice or rice cereal, Applesauce, Toast). Additional regimens can be suggested by your physician. Just ask.

Breast-fed infants should continue to breast-feed. If necessary to treat dehydration, balanced electrolyte solutions, such as Pedialyte or a similar solution, can be used between feedings. Breast-feeding mothers who have diarrhea should increase their intake of safe water and continue to breast-feed.

Symptoms that indicate the need to see a physician include fever greater than 102° F, bloody and/or watery stools, diarrhea that does not improve within twelve to twenty-four hours, and signs of dehydration such as decreased urination or dark urine, dry mouth, sunken eyes, and lethargy. Consult with a physician as soon as possible if your infant or child is not acting normal for his or her age or if your "gut feeling" tells you your child is sick.

If watery stools suggest the possible presence of cholera—a disease that can kill within hours—seek medical help immediately, especially for young children. Outbreaks of cholera can occur at any time in Africa, Asia, or South America.

If is not uncommon to have abdominal cramps accompanying diarrhea. A heating pad or hot water bottle (not too warm) may be helpful. Also skin irritation is common in diarrhea. Frequent diaper changes, an over-the-counter diaper cream, and warm baths may be soothing.

Ingesting contaminated food or water is the usual cause of infectious diarrhea. If you are planning to travel to a developing country or other area where the hygiene is questionable, ask your physician about both prevention and treatment of diarrhea for each member of the family. Different recommendations will be made, depending on the area to be visited and the age of the individual.

To help prevent diarrhea, always follow the safe food and water recommendations given at the beginning of this chapter. Additional suggestions include the following:

- Food is not the only source of bacterial contaminants. You and your children can pick up bacteria from such things as doorknobs and handrails. Everyone should wash their hands with soap and hot water before leaving a hotel room for meals.

- Avoiding recontamination on your way to the dining room is as important as washing your hands.

- When going down stairs where there is a handrail, train yourself and your children not to run hands down the handrail, thus certainly picking up any contaminating bacteria on the rail. Instead, you can simply place your hand outside of the rail, ready to grab it in case of a stumble. Carry children who are too small to do this or hold them by the hand.

- Before starting your trip, begin training your children to avoid touching surfaces such as door and faucet handles that can be contaminated in public places. Show them how to use the back of their hands, forearms, or a paper towel to avoid touching surfaces with the front of their hands and fingers that they use to pick up food.

Vomiting As with diarrhea, the main concern with vomiting is the risk of dehydration. The water and minerals required for replacement of body losses are similar to those required for diarrhea. However, liquids should be given in frequent and small amounts because they are more likely to be absorbed and less likely to be lost from recurrent vomiting. A physician should see all family members—especially infants and young children—who cannot stop vomiting, particularly if they appear to be dehydrated or have persistent pain.

Although vomiting is usually caused by an intestinal infection, it is also common in individuals with hepatitis or appendicitis. Individuals with symptoms of possible appendicitis must see a physician as soon as possible. Symptoms include low-grade fever, continuous abdominal (stomach) pain made worse by moving around, and little or no diarrhea. Otherwise, once a person stops vomiting, he or she usually can be slowly returned to a normal diet over a period of about twenty-four hours.

Be prepared by discussing diarrhea and vomiting with your physician before you go on your trip, especially if your child is under one year of age or has a chronic illness or recurrent intestinal problems. Infants and children can get sick quickly and dehydrate fast. If seen early and treated properly, they can also recover quickly.

Jet Lag

Crossing time zones upsets our brain's twenty-four-hour clock, called the *circadian rhythm,* and disturbs various body functions and routines, most noticeably those related to sleep and alertness, eating and digestion. The resulting mood disturbances, shortened attention span, poor concentration, and intestinal problems are upsetting to both children and adults and can get a family vacation off to a bad start or ruin a business trip.

People usually function best when they go to bed and get up at a set time each day. Thoughtful planning and anticipation can lessen the symptoms of jet lag. When applicable, consider these points:

- If time allows before your trip, gradually adjust your daily routine—the time you go to bed, get up, and eat—to your destination's schedule. If you are flying from, say, San Francisco to London or Tokyo, the change is greater than you can adjust to and still maintain your at-home work routine. However, adjusting halfway, or even a third of the way, will greatly lessen jet lag on your arrival at the distant point.

- If possible, schedule your arrival so that you have extra time to adjust to the time difference, especially if you will be required to make important decisions.

- Set your watch to the destination time while en route. This may help you adjust your eating and sleeping habits before you arrive.

- Minimize consumption of alcohol and exposure to tobacco smoke, which compound jet lag problems.

- If you must arrive in the morning, a short nap followed by a shower may increase your alertness.

- Try to sleep at the same time each night in the new time zone. If needed, try long hot showers or mild exercise to induce sleep. Over-the-counter sleep medications tend to cause decreased mental functioning the following day, and they lose their effectiveness within a few days.

- Avoid stimulants such as tea, coffee, hot chocolate, caffeine-containing soft drinks, and significant amounts of alcohol prior to bedtime. Conversely, a snack high in carbohydrates may be helpful.

- To help your circadian rhythm to adjust, get up at a reasonable time each morning, even if you have not had enough sleep, and eat protein-rich meals about the same time each day.

Because your twenty-four-hour clock is governed by sunlight, adjusting the times of your exposure to bright light and darkness can help readjust your circadian rhythm. When it is time to be awake, try to expose yourself to bright light, sunlight if possible, and when it is time to sleep, keep the sleeping area dark.

Many people swear by their own jet lag regimens, such as light exposure, jet lag diets, or medications such as melatonin or sleeping pills. Most travel physicians do not recommend melatonin for children, and safety issues are still being addressed. Research on jet lag is ongoing. Watch for new breakthroughs, decide what works the best for you, and always discuss your plans with your doctor.

Motion Sickness

Motion sickness is no joke to a sufferer of any age. A common reaction is, "First I thought I was going to die; then I was afraid I wouldn't." Motion sickness can happen in cars and planes, on boats, and even on amusement park rides. Children are especially susceptible to motion sickness, but because they are also very susceptible to suggestion, try to avoid talking about the condition before it happens.

Traveling in the front seat of a car is helpful, but for safety reasons it is not recommended for small children. If the car seats can be elevated enough for the child to see the horizon, this may overcome some of the problems related to riding in the backseat.

Before the initial dizziness or vague discomfort progresses to nausea and then to vomiting, try to find relief. Children concentrating on a game or drawing in the backseat, or adults reading while traveling in a car are more susceptible to motion sickness. The cure for this is simple: Stop reading and look outside at the most distant objects you can see until the symptoms subside.

Light snacking might help a child avoid motion sickness. (Saltine crackers are a favorite among sailors.) However, the idea of eating must appeal to the child; otherwise the light snack probably will not stay down.

People of any age are less likely to get motion sickness if they are exposed to circulating cool air rather than stagnant warm air. Over-the-counter medications such as Bonine and Dramamine are helpful to some people. Such medications can overstimulate some children, but the effects are usually sedating, which may make a long automobile trip more tolerable for children and their parents. Adolescents older than twelve years and adults may prefer the Transderm Scop, a prescription patch worn behind the ear, because it works for up to twelve hours. Although it can cause dry mouth and/or drowsiness, many people have fewer side effects from the patch than from oral medications for motion sickness. The patch should be worn only by the person for whom it is prescribed, as it can have serious side effects for some people. Follow application directions carefully and wash hands thoroughly after touching the patch.

Many families have found that pressure-point wristbands are effective in decreasing motion sickness. They are inexpensive and available in pharmacies and stores where travel goods are sold.

Nosebleeds

Nosebleeds are common when the skin inside the nose is dry—as can happen with a cold—and tend to be more frequent in cold weather. Nose-picking and injury can also cause frequent nosebleeds, especially during toddler years, when any small object is likely to be pushed into the nose. Keeping the nose moist with a saline spray will usually reduce the frequency of nosebleeds.

Many parents initially panic when a nosebleed comes on suddenly in a child, but nosebleeds are not usually serious and they stop spontaneously. A few pointers may be helpful:

- Leaning a little forward while seated is the best position. (Vomiting can occur if a child is allowed to lie down and the blood runs down the back of the throat.)

- Firm, continuous pinching of the soft part of the nose for ten minutes is best.

- Repeat these steps again if necessary.

Bleeding from the front of the nose through the nostril accounts for about 90 percent of nosebleeds and should stop with this treatment.

If the bleeding continues in the back of the nose, the person can usually tell, even though blood may not be coming out of the nostril. Contact a physician right away or evacuate the person immediately to seek medical help, because the bleeding cannot be stopped.

Recurrent nosebleeds can mean that a serious problem exists, such as concussion or facial fracture. Bleeding from both the front and the back of the nose may follow a trauma. Contact a physician immediately, as first aid may only be a problematic delay in treatment.

Overheating (Hyperthermia)

Overheating is a common, and potentially dangerous, problem in hot climates. If you are traveling to the tropics, try to stay in air-conditioned hotels. Avoid outdoor activities between 10:00 A.M. and 2:00 P.M. Wear heat-reflective clothing to help decrease heat exposure. The body protects itself from overheating by sweating, so dehydration is particularly dangerous. Here are some suggestions that will help you and your children avoid overheating:

- Fresh fruits and vegetables are a good source of salt and other minerals, but should be eaten only if they have been washed in safe water or if you can peel the fruits yourself. Talk with your doctor about taking salt tablets.

- Recognizing the early symptoms of overheating can help prevent serious problems such as heatstroke. If you or your child develop headaches, dizziness, muscle cramps, and/or general sluggishness, get out of the sun immediately, drink lots of fluids, bathe in cool water, and/or find cooler surroundings such as an air-conditioned automobile. If nothing else is available, find shade, lie down, drink fluids, and rest.

- Heat problems are aggravated by humidity because the moist air interferes with the cooling effects of evaporation of perspiration. Perspiration is a very effective mechanism for removing heat from the body, so hot, dry desert areas may be easier to tolerate than hot moist areas—as long as a person drinks lots of fluids to replace lost perspiration.

- In hot climates wear loose cotton clothing and a broad-brimmed hat. The hat should be designed to allow ventilation of air around the scalp.

Skin Rashes

Skin rashes are a common problem for the traveler. Dry skin can cause itching and be mistaken for ringworm. A lubricating cream and sunscreen are useful to prevent rashes, and an over-the-counter 1 percent hydrocortisone cream is helpful for treating red and itchy rashes after they develop. If itching is severe, an anesthetic cream that contains benzocaine and cool, wet towels or cloths are helpful to relieve the itching. If you have a chronic skin condition, check with your doctor.

Skin rashes are usually best treated by avoiding whatever causes them. Questions you should consider when trying to determine the cause of a skin rash include the following:

- When and where did the rash start? If the rash involves areas not covered by clothing, this suggests contact with a chemical or plant, or sun exposure, as the cause.

- Does it itch? Significant itching suggests an allergic cause.

- Does it seem to be associated with a particular travel activity or exposure to a medication whether taken orally or applied to the skin?

- Does it seem to be associated with a chemical, perfume, cream, or plant such as poison ivy?

- What makes the rash better, and what makes it worse?

- Are there any symptoms associated with the rash? Fever, sore throat, or swollen lymph glands suggest the rash is related to an infection.

Keeping the skin moist is key to preventing many skin problems. Dry, itchy, flaky, and cracking skin is likely to became inflamed when exposed to chemicals, such as those found in perfumes and soaps, that normally would not be irritating. Consider the following points to help protect the skin:

- Frequent swimming, scuba diving, and sun contact dry the skin, so be particularly alert to protecting the skin if you participate in these activities.

- Lubricating skin creams are best applied when the skin is moist, such as after a bath or shower.

- Soaps remove natural skin oils, so they are a common cause of dry skin and rashes. However, some soaps—Dove, Basis, and Lubriderm—are relatively gentle and are especially recommended for people with sensitive skin.

- Showering immediately after swimming can help wash rash-causing organisms, chemicals, and other irritants off the skin. This is particularly helpful after swimming in the tropics.

- Warm water encourages the growth of certain bacteria, so try to make certain that spas and hot tubs are properly sanitized. If not, avoid them.

Sleeplessness

Unfamiliar surroundings, beds, and time zones frequently cause sleep problems. Earplugs and eye masks may help convince your brain that it is time to sleep. A walk, a glass of warm milk, or a warm bath also can help. Many people have a favorite remedy.

Alcoholic refreshments may help people get to sleep, but they actually worsen sleep overall because people often awake within a few hours and cannot get back to sleep. Be particularly careful about imbibing alcohol if you are also taking medications, especially sleeping pills, because alcohol/drug interactions can be serious.

If you or your child has trouble sleeping, an over-the-counter antihistamine such as Benadryl or your favorite may be useful.

Try all medications prior to travel to be sure you don't experience the opposite of the intended effect or have a bad reaction.

Sunburn

Ultraviolet light from the sun causes sunburn. There is strong evidence that repeated severe sunburns in childhood are related to the later development of skin cancer in adults. According to the American Cancer Society, roughly 54,000 people will be diagnosed with skin cancer each year. Fair-skinned people are particularly at risk, but people of every complexion can sustain serious sunburn. Here are a few pointers for sun safety:

- Be aware that medications like antibiotics, antidepressants, and antihistamines increase a person's sensitivity to the sun.

- Use sunscreen with SPF 30 or more and reapply it after every session in the water, even if the sunscreen is supposed to be waterproof.

- Remember that "sunless" tanning lotions do not protect you from sunburn unless they have an SPF rating. SPF 30 is advisable.

- Wear a hat. A sunburned scalp not only is painful but can lead to dangerous overheating.

- Wear sunglasses. Even small children should wear sunglasses to protect their eyes from the cumulative damage of sun exposure.

- Cover up. The shade of an umbrella gives some protection, but only long sleeves and long pants truly guard limbs from the sun's rays. Snorkelers, who spend most of their time floating face down at the water's surface, should wear T-shirts while in the water to protect their backs from sunburn.

- Watch the tender spots. Ears, temples, neck, backs of knees, and tops of feet are easy to overlook when applying sunscreen and very painful when sunburned.

- Do not be fooled by overcast skies. A gray day is no guarantee of sun protection. Plenty of solar power burns through the overcast to scorch unprotected skin.

- Don't forget that sunburn typically looks and feels more intense after you get out of the sun. You may be sunburned even if your skin does not look red. Get out of the sun before you "see red."

- Keep an eye on the clock. Limit sun exposure altogether and try to minimize exposure during peak hours, usually between about 11:00 A.M. and 2:00 P.M., when the sun's rays are the most intense.

- Drink water. Even if you are not perspiring, you are losing body moisture to the sun's heat. Rehydrate early and often.

Upper and Lower Respiratory Infections

Colds and nasal congestion are common during travel largely because of exposure to many people in crowded conditions. Regular hand washing may significantly reduce the transmission of colds. Many travelers find that cold medications are effective but may have annoying side effects such as nervousness and sleeplessness. Medications such as Benadryl can be useful at night to improve sleep. Acetaminophen and aspirin (adults only) often help a person feel better, even if fever or headache is not present.

Being able to breathe through the nose really helps people sleep, so using nose drops or sprays just before bedtime is often worthwhile. Adults and older children can use a long-acting nasal spray such as Afrin. Children should use just one or two drops of a weaker preparation. Check this with your doctor. If used several times a day for more than a few days, chemical nose drops or sprays often cause irritation and rebound swelling of the nasal membranes. However, if these preparations are used only once daily at bedtime as a sleep aid, they can generally be used without side effects for seven to ten days.

Saline (saltwater) nose drops are used frequently, especially in infants, because they are less irritating to the nasal membranes. They are particularly helpful in infants for loosening secretions, which can then be aspirated (sucked out) with an infant nasal bulb (aspirator).

Coughs The most effective over-the-counter medication for suppressing an annoying cough is dextromethorphan, which is available in many different cough medications. Discuss with your doctor which one to use. Some people may become sleepy or excited from cold or cough medications, particularly those containing decongestants, so it is best to try those medications at home before traveling. Parents usually have a favorite antihistamine, decongestant, or cough medicine. Consult with a pediatrician before giving any medications to your child.

Medications such as diphenhydramine (Benadryl, for example) can cause drowsiness. They should not be used by anyone who will drive an automobile before the effects of the drug wear off. However, such medications may be useful for travelers, especially young children, because they may improve rest and decrease motion sickness.

Be sure you try all medications at home first. Occasionally, medications like Benadryl can cause a reaction opposite to the one expected.

Most of the time, without other complications, mild upper respiratory infections resolve themselves in one to two weeks. If a child is an infant and has allergies, asthma, or a chronic illness; is in day care or school; or has other siblings, he or she may be more susceptible to ear infections, bronchitis, or pneumonia. If upper respiratory symptoms seem to worsen, be alert to this possibility and obtain a medical evaluation at home or abroad.

General Health Concerns

If your child has a significant past medical history of ear infections; asthma; worrisome allergic reactions, such as anaphylaxis; a tendency toward motion sickness; diarrhea or constipation; or other chronic or potential health conditions, discuss your upcoming travel plans with your doctor at least three to four months prior to departure.

Have your child seen by a physician if he or she develops a significant temperature, has a change in normal behavior, continues to vomit and/or has diarrhea, has abdominal pain, has increased respiratory rate or heart rate, or has increasing wheezing. Be alert and vigilant, whether you are at home or abroad.

Most people travel again and again without incident, undisrupted by illness or injury. The protective vaccines, medications, and preventive and proactive care suggested in this chapter can guard you and your family against illness. But even more important, the information provided here can help you become more prepared, informed, and educated so that you will know how to handle common problems, how to get help if you need it, and have more peace of mind when traveling.

Chapter 4
What to Pack

As baggage restrictions and security checks increase for travelers everywhere, the words of the French writer Antoine de Saint-Exupéry seem ever more apt: "Those who would travel happily must travel light."

When you travel alone, you might be able to toss a few items into a carry-on bag and be on your way. Traveling with children, however, adds a new dimension to your packing and makes it ever more important that you choose carefully to accommodate the clothing and equipment needed for the climate and activities you will enjoy on your trip. (If you are packing for a camping trip, see Chapter 10.)

Let Your Children Do Their Own Packing

At least a couple of weeks before you leave on your trip, give each child an inexpensive but durable tote bag that is to be used for trips only. Explain that they will need to lift and carry their own bag, so they will have to make careful choices about what to bring.

Urge each child to make a personal packing list. This is a wonderful habit to adopt. Encouraging your children to take responsibility for packing their own things will help them become more independent and self-assured. It will also make your life easier.

Tell them to select toys and books they want to take on the trip and put them in their tote. This can eliminate tearful negotiations over which toys are taken and which are left behind. The child's checklist may also include:

- security blanket, stuffed animal, or other soothing object

- extra underwear and pants in case of accidents

- family photo or snapshot of a favorite pet

- disposable camera

You cannot expect small children to remember to pack all the things you consider essential. You will need to check over what they have packed, and you will certainly need to carry heavy or special items in your own suitcase.

Packing Tips

- Make a list, by person, of all the clothes and other items you plan to take, including how various items will be combined for each occasion. To be certain you have the right clothes, organize your list by date, showing which outfit each person will wear.

- Pack your suitcase several days in advance of your trip; if you do not, you are likely to find yourself packing in a rush at the last minute—a sure formula for taking too much and forgetting important items.

- Check current weather conditions and predictions for your destination before making final clothing choices. Plan for weather surprises—the summer rainstorm, icy air-conditioning, or a sudden midwinter thaw.

- Coordinate your wardrobe around a few colors and vary your outfits with accessories.

- Pack only what you can carry yourself. This is easier with two smaller suitcases. Wheeled cases are enormously helpful, but do not count on them if you are going to places with cobbled or unpaved roads or long flights of stairs.

- Bring zip-closure plastic bags, which are a great boon to packing. The heavier freezer weight bags come in an assortment of sizes suitable for everything from toiletries to undergarments to diapers to entire outfits for small children.

- Consider packing an extra duffel bag to carry your vacation purchases. If you do a lot of shopping on your trip, shipping your purchases home may be more practical than carrying them. Be sure to arrange with someone to receive your packages so that they—or the attempted-delivery notices—do not announce your absence.

- Wrap clothes in plastic bags or tissue paper to minimize wrinkling. Roll and fold the clothing and slip each day's outfit into a see-through plastic bag. Fit the plastic bags into your luggage. When you arrive at your first destination, hang only the items you will wear while there. Leave the rest in your suitcase to minimize repacking. The bags make everything visible; you will know what you have and where it is, and it will remain neatly folded.

- Check that all necessary travel documents, credit cards, and money will fit in concealed security pouches; that duplicate copies are in your checked luggage; and that a third set is in the hands of a reliable friend who is staying home.

Packing Checklists

Most seasoned travelers create a checklist to help them remember the items they will need on their trip. It is very frustrating to arrive at your destination and realize you have forgotten something. The time spent replacing needed items can cut into your enjoyment of the trip, and into your travel budget as well.

Make a three-part checklist—security pouch, carry-on bags, and suitcases—for each traveler, or use the following lists to make sure you have everything you need. If you are going camping or your trip involves sporting activities that require equipment, such as for skiing and scuba diving, make a separate list for each activity. A computer is the best way to keep track of your lists, but if you write them by hand, make sure to keep a copy so you will not have to start from scratch on your next trip!

Security Pouch

Your security pouch is always concealed inside your clothing. There are many different styles available. Find one that fits properly, is not visible or bulky with your typical clothing, and is not excessively hot for your destination.

Here's what goes in your security pouch:

- Passport

- Money. Keep most of your cash here. Carry a few small bills and only what you will need for the day in your wallet, purse, or pockets.

- Traveler's checks

- Credit cards. Keep only one in your wallet or purse.

- Tickets

- Home state and international driver's license (when you are not driving)—when you do get behind the wheel of an automobile, put your licenses in your wallet or purse.

Carry-on Bag

A carry-on bag packed with carefully selected items is your best protection if your luggage does not arrive where and when you do. It should also hold the items you will need to keep your family comfortable and occupied while you are in transit. Your children should pack their necessities in their own carry-on bags. Any extended—more than a weekend—trip with children will require more luggage than you can pack into carry-on bags.

Carry-on bags should include:

- Everything you really need to spend two nights without your checked bag-gage. Why two nights? Because it takes thirty-six hours for 98 percent of misrouted luggage to reach the aggrieved passengers. If medications are involved, prepare for the possibility that your bags could take three or more days to reach you.

- Extra underwear and nightclothes

- Your toiletries kit (see below)

- Prescription medications

- Travel alarm clock with a fresh battery

- Travel papers such as your itinerary, reservation confirmations and receipts, vouchers, and directions

- Photocopies of the first two pages of all passports in your party, plus copies of driver's licenses, vaccination/inoculation certificates, and trans-lated medical alert and medical insurance cards (with policy and phone numbers)

- Proof of auto insurance, even if you do not plan to drive. If you are going out of the country, contact your insurer to verify coverage.

- Copies of significant medical history, if pertinent

- Extra copies of medical and eyeglass prescriptions

- Addresses and telephone numbers for the American embassies or consulates where you are going, your physicians, and other important people

- Your complete travel medicine kit (see below) or a "mini" first-aid kit with bandages, antibiotic cream, moleskin for sore feet, SPF 30 (or higher) sunscreen, and lip balm

- Entertainment—books, magazines, games, toys—to keep you and your family occupied during plane flights and quiet times

- Your traveling office and crafts supplies, including pens, colored pencils, crayons, highlighters, scratch paper, Post-it notes, Scotch tape, and small notebooks

- Laptop computer, if appropriate

Toiletries

- Breath freshener or mouthwash

- Deodorant

- Disposable razor(s)

- Earplugs or eye shades, if you use them for travel

- Eyeglass repair kit

- Feminine hygiene items

- Foot powder, body powder

- Hair care supplies: shampoo, conditioner, comb, brush, clips

- Hand soap and dish soap to wash baby bottles, cups, spoons

- Makeup

- Medications in their original containers

- Moisturizing lotion

- Nail care items

- Rubber drain stopper for hand laundry; a flat round stopper will work in most sinks and tubs

- Skin care lotions, sunscreen, lip balm

- Tissues, towelettes, cotton balls, swabs

- Toothbrushes, toothpaste, dental floss

- Waterless hand-washing lotion

Checked Luggage

- An extra copy of your packing checklist. Use your checklist not only when you pack the first time, but every time you repack to make sure nothing is left behind.

- Copies of travel papers, such as your itinerary, tickets, reservation confirmations and receipts, vouchers, directions, packing lists, and a list of traveler's checks serial numbers. Carry the serial numbers separate from the checks so you will not lose both if a handbag or suitcase is lost or stolen.

- Spare set of sunglasses and eyeglasses or contact lenses and lens cleaner

- Undergarments

- Sleepwear and bathrobe, including wet-dry slippers for shower wear

- One outfit for each kind of occasion you expect to encounter. This is where most overpacking is done, so examine your choices carefully.

- Inexpensive, lightweight accessories that can make the same outfit look entirely different: scarves, shawls, beads, silk flowers, hats

- Shoes, stuffed with socks

- Gear appropriate to the climate you will encounter, for example, overcoat or parka with hood, cap, mittens or gloves, scarf

- Sports equipment such as snorkels and masks, fins, workout clothes, swimsuits, ski gloves

- Rain gear appropriate to your destination: umbrella, galoshes or rubbers to go over your shoes, raincoat. If you are not likely to encounter rainy weather, consider carrying a lightweight plastic poncho for emergencies.

- Flashlight and extra batteries

- Sewing kit: needles, thread, scissors, safety pins

- Bag for dirty laundry

- Travel alarm clock

- Blow-dryer. Many hotels and motels supply dryers in every room; others may have dryers available on request.

- Travel iron. As with blow-dryers, you will find that many hotel rooms come equipped with irons and ironing boards.

- Safety equipment, such as night-light(s), electric socket covers

- Extra duffel bag for purchases

Your Child's Suitcase

- Two or more outfits for each day of travel, including shirts, pants, and underwear. The amount of clothing you take will be dictated by the activities you have planned, your child's age and mobility, and your access to laundry facilities.

- Extra underwear and socks

- "Dress-up" clothes as appropriate to your itinerary

- Lightweight vest, sweater, sweatshirt, or jacket. Drawstrings in hoods can strangle or choke a child if they are caught in play equipment, a car door, or elsewhere. Look for clothing that uses snaps or other pull-apart closures.

- Heavy jacket with hood

- Mittens and knit cap

- Rain gear and rain boots

- Swimsuits

- Pajamas and slippers

- Shoes for various activities

- Protective gear, such as kneepads, helmet, and wrist and elbow guards

- Toiletries including hairbrush, comb, and toothbrush. Adolescents can carry their own shampoo, toothpaste, mouthwash, and other personal care items; put toiletries for younger children in your own kit.

Assembling an Effective Travel Medicine Kit

Begin gathering your travel medicine kit as soon as your trip is confirmed. Organize it in a small but sturdy, preferably waterproof, bag. Tuck in a few paper towels. Consider taking it in your carry-on luggage to reduce the possibility of loss.

Include all the medications family members normally take. Carry them in their original bottles to ease your way through customs, and carry a supply that will last several days beyond your planned itinerary, in case you should be delayed. Replenishing your medications in foreign countries may be difficult or undesirable.

Organize each person's medications in a zip-closure plastic bag and print his or her name on the bag with an indelible marker. Always carry copies of your prescriptions separate from your travel medicine kit in case the kit is lost.

It's also a good idea to bring with you emergency numbers for all your family physicians and copies of significant medical histories, as appropriate.

You may not need all the items listed here or you may need special equipment that is not on this list; the intention is to provide a general-purpose checklist that applies to different kinds of trips. Bear in mind that any first-aid kit is only as effective as the person using it, so it would be smart to take a first-aid course or refresher course before you travel with your children. Your kit should include the following:

- Ace bandage
- Acetaminophen (adult and children's strengths)
- Antibacterial ointment
- Antibacterial soap
- Antidiarrheal medication
- Anti-itch ointment
- Antiseptic wipes
- Bags, plastic, in assorted sizes
- Bandages and bandage tape
- Bandana, sling-sized
- Calamine lotion
- Cotton balls or pads
- Cotton swabs for ears
- Dental floss
- Denture adhesive
- Diaper-rash ointment
- Ear- and eyedrops/ointments
- Epi-kit (epinephrine for allergic reactions to bee stings)
- Extra eyeglasses or contact lenses. Include a copy of the lens prescription.

- Handbook of poisonous plants specific to your destination

- Hemorrhoid medication

- Hydrogen peroxide

- Insect repellant with DEET. Read directions and use with care.

- Instant cold compress

- Laxatives

- Lip balm

- MedicAlert bracelets and medical information summary

- Medications. Keep all prescription medications in their original containers; carry copies of prescriptions separately.

- Moist towelettes

- Moisturizing cream

- Moleskin/corn pads

- Mosquito netting with fasteners (or safety pins, if necessary)

- Needle and tweezers for splinters. Airline regulations require that these be checked with your luggage, not carried onboard.

- Rubber gloves

- Rubbing alcohol

- Scissors. These must be packed in checked luggage for air travel.

- Snakebite kit

- Sunscreen rated 30 SPF or greater. Although avoiding sunburn is paramount, you may also want to include a salve or spray to reduce the discomfort of sunburn, such as an aloe vera gel.

- Sunglasses with UV-protection-rated lenses

- Syrup of ipecac, to induce vomiting in case a child accidentally imbibes some poisonous product; use only with physician's instructions.

- Tecnu, to wash off poison oak or poison ivy resin

- Thermometer. To convert Celsius to Fahrenheit, multiply degrees Celsius by 9, divide the result by 5, and add 32.

- Tongue depressor

- Toothpaste and toothbrushes

- Vitamins

- Waterless hand-washing lotion

- Whistle, for emergencies

Items Necessary When Traveling with an Infant

For any mode of transportation, take a good supply of premoistened wipes or even a wet washcloth in a plastic bag.

By Car

- Baby food, plastic spoon, formula, juice

- Pacifiers

- Diaper bag, disposable diapers, changing pads

- Nursing pads, burp pads, bib

- Bathing supplies: towel, washcloth, soap, shampoo, powder, lotions, creams

- Bottle warmer, bottles, caps, nipples

- Car seat

- Child wrist handholder

- Medications, vitamins, thermometer

- Nail clippers

- Night-light

- Small plastic bowl with lid and training cup

By Sea

On a cruise you will unpack only once, and luggage limitations are more liberal than on other forms of transportation. Consider taking all the equipment for land travel suggested above plus:

- Portable crib or playpen. Some cruise lines can supply both, but do not count on it unless you have confirmed that one will be available.

- Waterproof crib sheets

- Crib-size blankets

- Potty seat

- Umbrella stroller, if desired

- Zip-closure plastic bags in various sizes

By Air

- Baby food, plastic spoon, formula, juice

- Pacifiers

- Diaper bag, disposable diapers, changing pads

- Nursing pads, burp pads, bib

- Premoistened wipes

Luggage Suggestions

Choose well-made, lightweight luggage with sturdy locks and built-in wheels. Choosing the right luggage can help prevent back problems. Two smaller suit-cases are better than one large suitcase you cannot easily lift. Put identification tags on both the outside and inside of each case and use a business address, if possible. And, most important, never leave your bags unattended!

- Do not count on finding porters standing by ready to assist you everywhere you go. Travel as efficiently as possible.

- Shoulder bags are very practical, but remember to give your shoulders a rest. Do not use just one shoulder to carry a bag; shift from shoulder to shoulder. This will prevent a constant heavy weight on one side that could result in shoulder or back pain. Two small shoulder bags are ideal for some travelers.

- The great popularity of backpacks has spread beyond students. Some back-packs are made especially for storage in airline overhead compartments. Many are available in stylish luggage materials and colors. They distribute the weight evenly across your shoulders and can be very convenient if you plan on extensive walking as part of your trip. Pack the heaviest objects so they ride close to your back. Do not place important documents or money in your pack because backpacks are especially vulnerable to pickpockets.

- Luggage with wheels may tempt you to take more than you can carry. Resist the temptation; if a wheel breaks, you will be lugging a heavy suitcase around.

- Some travelers prefer fold-up pull-carts so they can transport heavy loads easily. Test carts first to see that the handles are at a proper height for you, the wheels are sturdy, and the carts go up and down stairs easily.

Part II

Travel Challenges
and Solutions

Chapter 5
Other Travel Situations

Pregnant Parents on the Road

No car seats, no diapers, and no formula yet—it is the perfect time to travel, right? Maybe. Or maybe not. Before you make your plans, consider your condition and your destination. Start by asking yourself these questions:

- Are you knowledgeable about the complications of pregnancy?

- Have you talked with your doctor about your travel plans?

- Is adequate medical care available where you are going? Are adequate hospitals available if complications occur?

- Do you have any predisposing conditions or prior pregnancy problems that can only be treated close to home?

- Does your travel require vaccinations that could put your fetus at risk? Medications to treat and prevent conditions encountered by travelers may cause unpleasant—or potentially dangerous—side effects for pregnant women.

- Does your health insurance cover you, your delivery, and your newborn at your destination?

Call your airline to find out its requirements for flying when pregnant. Many airlines require a medical note if a woman wants to fly within a month of her due date and may not allow her to board if she cannot produce a doctor's letter. Be sure to make several photocopies of your doctor's letter. Keep the original and give the copies to airline clerks; you may need several before your round-trip is completed.

Although not all airlines require proof that the mother-to-be has her obstetrician's clearance to fly, common sense dictates that it should be obtained if you look pregnant. Get the clearance in writing even if your departure airline does not require it. Unexpected developments may force you to return on a different airline that does require written medical clearance, which may be difficult to get once you are away from home.

Women with health problems and women who are at risk of pre-term labor or have placental abnormalities should not fly when pregnant. For healthy women having a low-risk pregnancy, flying during the second trimester will be the safest and most comfortable. At that stage, any nausea they may have endured in their first trimester is probably past and they are not yet suffering the fatigue that often accompanies the final trimester.

Mothers-to-be should take steps to increase their comfort by avoiding gas-producing foods and carbonated drinks before and during the flight. High altitude tends to increase discomfort from bloating and gas. This problem is more acute for pregnant women because the expanded uterus puts pressure on the stomach and other organs.

Obstetricians generally advise pregnant women not to travel more than 300 miles from home after the twenty-eighth week of pregnancy. The American College of Obstetricians and Gynecologists (ACOG) published an official opinion in December 2001 advising that during a completely normal pregnancy domestic air travel is safe through the thirty-sixth week and international air travel through the thirty-fifth week. As of this writing, the Federal Aviation Administration does not require an emergency landing if a passenger goes into labor during a flight.

Ask for an aisle seat to make it easier to walk around and visit the rest room. However, pregnant women should remain in their seats as much as possible to avoid the possibility of falling in case of turbulence. Stay seated and buckled up, wearing the belt low. You can exercise in your seat by rotating your feet, by pushing against the floor with your toes and raising your heels, and by pressing one hand against the other. Such exercise will lessen swelling and boost blood circulation.

Here are some more points to remember if you must travel while pregnant:

- Unless your home is in a high altitude, avoid destinations above 8,000 feet.

- The effectiveness of your immune system may be significantly reduced by pregnancy. Use extra care to avoid infections.

- Some vaccines, motion-sickness medications, and other medications can cause serious problems to pregnant travelers.

- Avoid traveling to regions where infectious diseases such as malaria are prevalent. Malaria is more severe during pregnancy. Mosquito and other insect bites may expose you—and your unborn baby—to malaria, dengue fever, Lyme disease, and other insect-transmitted conditions. Drugs and topical repellents may be risky as well. If possible, defer your travel to third-world countries—especially those with malaria—until after your pregnancy.

- Travel only to countries and cities where you can be sure of obtaining first-class medical care.

- Be cautious about entering saunas, hot tubs, swimming pools, and the like. Never do so unless you will be able to bathe afterwards.

- Break up long automobile trips with frequent stops so you can walk around.

- Take ample supplies of your own vitamins and medications.

- If carsickness was a problem even before you became pregnant, consider postponing your travels.

- If you are in an auto accident—even if you walk away unhurt—consult a physician.

Whether you stay home or hit the road, make your plans carefully and do everything possible to keep yourself—and your baby—safe and comfortable.

Traveling with an Infant

If you did not have a compelling reason for taking on the complexities of traveling with an infant, you might not do it. But in many ways, traveling with a tiny one is easier than traveling with an older child: The little person is completely under your control. Rambunctious toddlers and sub-teens, on the other hand, are fast on their feet and may trot off at any moment.

As with any travel, vacationing with your infant could be a dream vacation or a nightmare. But if you are healthy, strong, willing to plan ahead, and can "go with the flow," you can equip yourself to manage any problems and enjoy a welcome respite from the routines of home. Here are some things to think about as you plan your trip:

- Be sensible with your travel plans. Are mom, dad, and baby ready?

- Test your travel-worthiness by starting with short trips.

- Be prepared with baby equipment, but travel as light as possible.

- If your infant is fussy or seems sick, do not go.

- If you are breast-feeding, decide in advance how you will attend to this essential function of mothering. Bring a scarf, shawl, or handkerchief to serve as a modesty cover. (Breast-feeding protects your infant against food- and waterborne diseases as it keeps the child calm, fed, and hydrated. Be sure to increase your own intake of fluids, and be aware that travel may disrupt your milk output.)

- Be careful taking your infant into areas of extreme temperatures.

- If you rely on electric appliances for heating, cooling, or sterilizing, make a backup plan in case the power goes out.

- If you do not feel comfortable with a baby-sitter at home, do not plan to use one when you are traveling.

- Before you put them to use, be sure that car seats, playpens, and strollers are safe.

- When you fly, try to stay away from sick passengers.

- When you book your flight, check with the airline regarding its seat requirements for infants.

- Children under three are more at risk for traveler's diarrhea than are older children or adults.

- Talk to your child's doctor about any concerns you might have.

- Test all equipment with your baby before you leave home. Make sure that baby carriers fit you and the baby properly and are comfortable.

- Also test lotions (sunscreen, for example) and, if practical, medications, before you leave home. On the road is not a good place to experience a bad reaction.

- You may have to carry your infant more than you anticipated. Pack your favorite—and well-tested—walking shoes.

Knowledge is the key to successful travel. If you are prepared and realistic, you can have a great trip with your infant.

Twins and Multiples

If travel is complicated by the presence of one child, it is certainly further complicated by the presence of two or more children. The situation becomes even more demanding when the children are twins or other multiples (triplets, quadruplets). Although nontwin siblings who are very close in age are not technically multiples, it is not unusual for a mother to be caring for two children in diapers. From a travel perspective, children so close in age present many of the same challenges—and rewards—as multiples. If traveling with multiples is on your itinerary, allow two to three extra weeks in your planning and consider the following suggestions:

- Tell your travel agent. Be prepared to explain the ages, travel experience, and special needs of each child.

- If you are booking your own reservations, inform the airline or other transportation company that you are traveling with multiples. Purchase a seat for each child and see if you can secure bulkhead seating, which is slightly more spacious and a bit more removed from other passengers.

- If you will be staying in a hotel, request cribs or other special equipment well in advance. Be sure to verify that the hotel has the size and number of cribs, high chairs, or other gear you will need.

- Pack complete outfits for each child in small, see-through bags.

- Let each child choose a favorite toy to take along. Don't expect multiples to share a single toy.

- When you have multiple infants or toddlers, consider renting equipment at your destination rather than carrying everything with you, but don't forget you will need car seats for travel to and from the airport.

- If possible, put an adult in charge of each child. Combined with unique clothing for each child, this can help to minimize the curious stares, uninvited touching, and continual photo requests that are likely when the children are seated together in a twin or triplet stroller. Change the arrangement periodically to give everyone a break.

- Check strollers onto the plane at the departure gate rather than with checked baggage so you can pick them up immediately on arrival.

- Call ahead for an airport electric tram to transport you to connecting flights or to the baggage claim area if it is a long distance away.

- Arrange your schedule so that each child has some time alone with you, without a sibling.

- Multiples attract a great deal of attention, so be sure to attend to the needs of your other children, who may feel left out or shortchanged.

- Expect to be tired and plan for rest time.

With the increase in the number of twin and multiple births, travel with multiples is more common, and airlines, hotels, and restaurants are becoming more skilled at accommodating them. Plan ahead, get plenty of rest, and don't forget your camera!

Traveling with Another Family

When planning a vacation, consider whether you and your children would find greater enjoyment by sharing your vacation with another family. For single parents, this can be a terrific way to ease some of the problems of travel with children and also to enjoy being with adult companions.

Before you consider traveling with other people, get to know them well. Rather than jumping into a two-week vacation, try a weekend trip first. If you can't enjoy a weekend in their company, you can count on being miserable on a longer trip. Be sure that both your families have the same expectations.

Be clear about the handling of finances. Any confusion in this area can result in misunderstanding or resentment during the trip and afterwards. If the other party is evasive about how costs will be shared, you may be making a mistake in including them in the trip. Trust your instincts, and do not count on figuring it out "later."

Try to have as many details as possible worked out before you travel. For example, how will you handle planning, cooking, cleaning up, leading activities, and so on? Instead of assuming "they should just know" that you want help, talk about this before the trip, and ask for assistance before it becomes an issue. Discuss also the sharing of duties and which activities you will enjoy either together or separately. If your trip includes car travel, talk about how the driving duty will be shared.

Finally, talk about schedules. Find out whether children have the same bedtimes. Also ask in advance whether your companions are typically early, on time, or late. This is a common source of stress among travelers, and knowing what to expect will be very helpful.

Your vacation will be more satisfactory if you know in advance that the children enjoy each other's company and are close in age. Equally important is that the adults find each other congenial.

Note: Discipline varies among parents. Be aware of this and respect each other's discipline styles.

Taking Your Child's Friend Along

Taking your child's friend along can make the trip more fun for everyone—or it can be a nightmare. Unfortunately, such a nightmare can continue long after the trip is over, leading to acrimony between the children and the families.

When faced with the decision of whether to include your child's friend on a trip, consider not only the child's personality but also that of his or her parents. Some more practical considerations include the following:

- Will the other parents give you written authorization to secure medical treatment if your child-guest requires it?

- Does your child's friend have any allergies or other medical conditions or require medication?

- Will your insurance cover his or her medical expenses, or do the child's parents have medical coverage? If not, who will pay?

- Can you be sure the child-guest will accept your guidance and behave according to your concept of acceptable conduct? Does he or she observe any special behavioral rules?

- What if the child-guest's behavior threatens to ruin the entire family's vacation? Is he or she old enough to fly home alone if that becomes necessary?

- Have you discussed any expectations about money beforehand? If you invite your child's friend on the trip, you should probably plan to pay his or her expenses. Under some circumstances (say, a team trip) it might be appropriate for the child's parents to pay for transportation and other costs.

Again, a weekend sleepover or a few days out of town can give you a good idea of how your child's friend fits in with your family and responds to your directions. If short-term visits are successful, then advance to longer trips.

Pets and Children on the Road

If you are looking for relaxation on your vacation, consider putting your pets in a kennel until you return. Some people think that taking their children along doubles the stress of traveling; taking pets doubles it again. Before you commit to taking the family dog along, visualize yourself shepherding kids and pet through busy terminals.

Also do your research. For example, Hawaii and Alaska have strictly enforced laws about admitting dogs, cats, or other animals. Many hotels refuse to allow pets in guest rooms. Some provide outside kennels but most make no provision at all for pets. Call ahead and make sure that every place you plan to stay at will accept your pet under conditions that are acceptable to you. The auto club and several on-line services publish guides to pet-friendly inns, motels, hotels, resorts, and other types of lodgings in the United States and Canada.

If you have decided to take your children along on a business trip or a vacation and are thinking about also taking one or more pets, the decisive question should be, "Will taking the pets endanger my child?" Ushering children and pets through busy terminals can distract you long enough to lose sight of one or both. Consider the value of not being outnumbered by your charges. When thrust into strange circumstances, a dog is even less predictable than a small child.

As you are deciding whether it is safe to take your pet on a trip, consider these factors:

- Type of trip. Public transportation of all kinds can pose special problems.

- Animal diseases. You might run into rabies-control problems at your destination.

- Behavior of both children and pets. Can you control all of them with leash or voice commands?

- Stress. Can you handle the added anxieties?

If you have never taken your children and pets on a trip, ease into it with short excursions in your own car where you have the greatest control. Make sure that you can rely on good behavior and are ready to handle the challenges of public travel before you commit to train, aircraft, or ship. Once committed, it may be difficult or expensive to change your plans if you think better of it.

Traveling with kids and pets is most convenient when done by car. This permits frequent stops for boredom relief and exercise. Travel on public conveyances may require stowing your pet with the baggage. In this case, both you and your pet may be happier if the animal stays at home.

Be aware that when crossing the border between the United States and Canada—both ways—you must produce a health certificate signed by a licensed veterinarian to prove that your pet is rabies-free. Special rules apply if you are entering Canada through Newfoundland. Contact the Canadian Embassy at 501 Pennsylvania Avenue NW, Washington, D.C. 20001; Web site: www.canadianembassy.org.

Travel with pets outside the continental United States poses an entirely new set of problems, such as coping with quarantines and having proof of vaccination against rabies. Inquire well in advance about documentation, permits, vaccinations, and quarantines required in each country you plan to visit.

Different rules apply to birds and other types of pets. Research the rules in advance or leave your pets at home.

When Your Child Has to Fly Solo

There are many reasons why a child might need to make an unaccompanied flight. If this happens in your family, here are some points to consider:

- Contact the airline to see whether your child is old enough to make the proposed trip unaccompanied by an adult.

- Choose nonstop flights, if possible. If the trip requires a change of planes, make sure this is also acceptable to the airlines.

- If you have reliable friends or relatives living near the connecting airport, consider asking one of them to be on hand to usher your child through the connection.

- Check on pickup at the destination.

    o Will a flight attendant accompany your child off the aircraft?

    o Will the airline require identification before turning the child over to the person meeting the flight?

- Give your child written instructions on what to do in case of a delayed connecting flight.

- If possible, give the child a cell phone that will also work where he or she is going.

- Consider what will happen if a connecting flight is cancelled, and devise a plan to deal with it.

- On departure, take your solo flier to the airport; do not leave the airport until the aircraft takes off.

- Once the plane is off the ground, call the people meeting the child and give them the estimated arrival time.

- Your children should never wear anything on their outer clothing that gives their name: no tags or names embroidered on clothing. The wrong kind of person can gain their trust by calling them by name.

- You will not be able to board the aircraft with your child since you are not a passenger on that flight. Arrange beforehand to contact one of the flight's cabin attendants who will take charge of getting your child(ren) seated aboard the aircraft.

- Make sure that whoever picks up your child at the other end is a reliable person, preferably someone the child knows. Make sure he or she uses the "family code word" to greet your child.

- Tell your child how to call a flight attendant in case any problems arise.

Your Secret Vacation Spot: Home

You didn't plan a deception, it just happened: You were out of town and came home a day earlier than expected. Your friends and coworkers didn't know you were home. You didn't have to be anywhere or do anything. The phone didn't ring. So you did something you never do at home: nothing.

Maybe you have experienced the luxury of that unexpected one-day-at-home vacation—or maybe you can imagine it. Either way, you have captured the essence of a unique and rewarding plan for your next vacation: Stay home.

As with any vacation, your at-home time will benefit from advance planning. And whether you want a romantic hideaway or a family retreat, you can design the atmosphere and events to meet your needs. Here are a few tips to consider before you "go":

- Mark your vacation on your calendar and make sure nothing mundane is planned for that time—no dental appointments, no car pools, and no meetings.

- Well in advance, start watching the local paper for concerts, sporting events, and other activities you would enjoy but do not usually attend. Buy tickets.

- Talk about the things that really define a vacation for you. Fill in the blank: "I've always wanted to _____." Some people want nothing more than endless hours reading in a hammock; others want to see, learn, and explore. Some want to be pampered; others want to be left alone. How can you bring those elements home?

- Consider renting equipment that you might enjoy if you were traveling away from home: a convertible, a chauffeured limousine, a motor scooter, a boat.

- Food is an important part of your vacation. Depending on whether you are dreaming of an at-home rustic camp or a luxurious resort, you may want to eat some meals in and some out. Plan meals and stock up on supplies ahead of time. You don't want to spend your vacation at the supermarket! Make a list of restaurants you would like to try. Remember, this is your vacation, so don't do ordinary things. Consider home delivery or even hiring a cook to prepare special meals in your home. You may want to enroll in a cooking workshop at a local college or culinary school and make that a sidelight of your vacation.

- Post your "to do" list and on it write "Things We *Won't* Do on Our Vacation."

- Camping? Why not? Pitch the tent. Build a campfire. Roast marshmallows. Tell ghost stories. Sing songs.

- Take pictures. Make sure everyone in the house has a camera and film (disposables are great) to record your vacation memories. Work on your vacation scrapbook and think up funny captions for your photos.

- Send postcards. Buy local picture postcards or make your own.

- What about mementos? What kind of gift item truly represents your hometown? Perhaps it's a food product, a T-shirt, or a piece of art. Whether you are buying a gift for someone else or for yourself, find something that captures the place you spent your vacation.

- Do something physical, but make sure it is not what you do every other day of the year. Do not go to your usual gym. Explore a park. Hire a private trainer or coach to come to the house. Go horseback riding. Take scuba lessons.

- Plan a few separate activities—for kids and adults. Do not spend every second together. It is easy to slip into routine behavior when you're vacationing at home. Make sure you have enough plans to keep your days fresh.

- Be a tourist. Take a tour of your hometown. See the highlights from a visitor's perspective.

- Treat yourself. Indulge in a relaxing massage, facial, pedicure, and sauna.

- Turn off your cell phone. Ignore your e-mail. Don't call the office. Don't set the alarm clock. You are on vacation.

- Let someone else clean up the mess. If washing dishes and doing the laundry is not part of your ideal vacation, consider booking a cleaning service to come in and handle the "dirty work" while you relax.

You do not have to leave home to have a vacation, you just need to vacate ordinariness. Be creative. Have fun planning and plan to have fun. Who knows, after a vacation at home, you may find yourself enjoying your home more than ever.

Chapter 6
Grand Trips
with Grandparents

Vacations with grandparents can be rewarding for everyone. They offer opportunities for closer bonds between generations, and bring new perspectives to the familiar cast of characters on family trips.

If the children's grandparents are vigorous and compatible, including them in your travel plans can be a tremendous help. Bringing your best and most dependable baby-sitters along means that Mom can get a few precious and well-deserved hours away from the relentless responsibilities of motherhood every vacation day. Equally important, this means the parents can spend a little carefree time together as they did before the children came.

If you are a grandparent, there are many ways to approach a multigenerational vacation and to make sure it is enjoyable and safe for everyone.

Such vacations can take different forms: One or both grandparents may take a grandchild on a trip, parents may include grandparents on family trips, a child may be invited for a stay-over at the grandparents' home, or grandparents and children may take day trips near home. Planning the right vacation depends on the age, health, interests, and capabilities of both grandparents and children. The parents, of course, must be ready to let their children take whatever trip is proposed.

Planning the Multigenerational Trip

When a traveling family includes people from more than two generations, a considerable difference in fitness is possible. Small children or physically inactive grandparents may be unable to do things that young adults take in stride. Compare the relative fitness of each member of the travel group to the physical demands that will be involved before settling on a trip's activities.

In the absence of physical problems, considerations for health, safety, packing, and planning are much the same for parents as for grandparents. However, unless the grandparents live with the grandchildren, they need to make a special effort to share these important steps with the children. If they live nearby, planning sessions are easier, but even at a distance, phone, fax, e-mail, and U.S. mail can work very well.

Any time you consider leaving your children in the care of their grandparents, your first consideration must be the welfare of your children. The suitability of your parents to assume control of your children has to be weighed on the same scale you would use for any other baby-sitter.

If you know of any physical, mental, or emotional reasons why your children will not be safe when alone with one of your grandparents, make sure that situation does not arise. At the same time, be as kind as possible to the grandparent involved.

If both sets of grandparents are healthy, suitable, and available to travel, choosing only one pair to join you on a premium trip may result in hard feelings that last a long time. Avoid the choice: Take no grandparents at all or divide the trip into two parts.

Before subjecting grandparents or kids to too many surprises, here are a few suggestions:

- Make the planning part of the journey. Grandparents and grandchildren will learn a great deal about each other as they plan their vacation. Use books, magazines, maps, newspaper travel sections, and the Internet to pre-explore your destination. Let children make suggestions and express preferences, with the understanding that they may not be able to do everything on their wish list.

- Make sure everyone is prepared for the unexpected. Travel is full of surprises, no matter who is involved. Travelers should be ready to change their plans if necessary, and to understand that they can still have a good time.

- Test for roadworthiness. Grandparents may be nostalgic about their youthful travels, but such notions do not ensure successful vacations today. Whatever the vacation plan, schedule a "mini" version—one day, one night, not too far from home—to let grandparents and grandchildren see whether they enjoy each others' company.

- Consider sending one grandchild at a time. A trip alone with Grandma is a special treat. A trip with all the siblings is likely to be a lot like every other day, just moved to a new location. A single child will get abundant attention, plus the child left behind will be more available for "quality time" with parents at home. If each child can look forward to his or her special trip, that child won't feel cheated if this is his or her turn to stay home. Besides, one child is probably more manageable for grandparents in terms of stamina. If there are two grandparents, they might want to consider inviting along the grandchild's friend.

- Explain the rules. The lucky grandchild may get to stay up a little later or have an extra scoop of ice cream, but grandparents should still be prepared to honor the important rules set by parents. This means having a frank discussion before making any plans. Topics should include dietary restrictions, bedtime, money, homework, medications, and allergies, to name just a few. Be sure that Grandpa knows if your child sleepwalks, wets the bed, or has nightmares. Talk about swimming skills. If your child has any special needs, carefully review how these might affect travel plans. Put everything in writing, along with medical insurance policy numbers and phone numbers for doctors.

- Provide a written (and notarized) document that clearly gives your permission for the grandparent(s) to travel with, care for, and secure medical treatment for your children. Children and grandparents should be fully identified by name in the document. Send one copy with the grandparents, keep one at home, and give a third copy to your children's physician.

You want your child's vacation to be memorable, but such memories should not come at the price of exhausting the physical resources or goodwill of grandparents. Plan short trips at first; travel time can be lengthened on future vacations, once grandparents and grandchildren have shown themselves to be worthwhile traveling companions.

Before Committing to a Trip with Your Grandchildren, Ask Yourself These Questions

- Have we taken short trips with our grandchildren's parents along? Do we feel comfortable taking the children without their parents?

- Raising our own children involved dealing with one generation gap. Traveling alone with grandchildren involves coping with two generation gaps. Can all of us handle it?

- Do the grandchildren have a favorable or antagonistic attitude toward the proposed trip with us but without their parents?

- What are our financial, and especially our physical and emotional, limitations?

- Is the destination—its climate, activities, opportunities, and hazards—appropriate for the ages of our grandchildren?

- Does where we will be going have programs for children?

- How do we feel about taking on this responsibility?

- What is involved in thoroughly preparing for the proposed trip?

- Do our grandchildren relate well to us? Will they obey our instructions?

- Have we taken short trips with the parents along to familiarize ourselves with the reality of managing their children?

- Have we looked into the many excellent programs for grandchildren traveling with their grandparents?

- Do our methods of discipline harmonize with those of our grandchildren's parents?

Before Taking a Trip with Your Grandchildren, Review These Considerations

- What is the best trip to take with our grandchildren—long or short? Local or international?

- Have we prepared a first-aid kit and taken a class in CPR?

- Do we know the important health hazards for children of different ages?

- Do we have written authority from the parents to secure necessary medical treatment for the children?

- What modes of transportation are available to us and which do we prefer?

- Would we consider taking our grandchild's friend along? At what age?

- What provisions must we make to keep us and our grandchildren happy and safe while traveling?

- How can we plan a trip that will be interesting to children of different ages?

Assuming the Parental Role: Advice for Grandparents

Your first duty is to minimize your own problems and risks so you will have more time and energy for the parental role. Consider acting on these recommendations:

- Get your doctor's permission to begin a regular exercise program to improve your strength, flexibility, and cardiovascular system. This will also have a favorable impact on your immune system.

- Condense bulky medical data into a compact form so you can keep the vital information with you on your travels.

- Organize your gear so you can travel light. Start on this as early as possible. Decisions made under last-minute time pressures will result in you lugging more weight around.

- Take care of your back. Consider special exercises to strengthen back muscles.

- If you will be flying or going to high altitude areas, see your ophthalmologist if you have a history of retinal disease.

- Check on your immunization needs well ahead of your departure date. Some immunizations take time to become effective.

- Check with your physician to see if you need medication to prevent malaria. In some countries, strains of malaria resist traditional malaria medications. Discuss this with your physician or a specialist in travel medicine.

- Know your limitations. Think about your stamina, your physical and mental flexibility, your walking ability, and your sleep requirements. Consider your phobias and allergies, if any.

- Travel in groups. Avoid night travel as much as possible.

- Consider going on organized tours. They are generally far less stressful.

- Prepare your first-aid kit for the trip as early as possible. A well-stocked first-aid kit is not just useful for travel; it is also a valuable asset to have at home.

- Do you have a MedicAlert bracelet? Do you need one because of chronic conditions or allergies? If so, don't delay obtaining one.

- Look into obtaining insurance to cover the cost of medical evacuation by air.

- See a physician regularly and discuss your travel plans, especially if you have chronic conditions or have recently suffered an injury or acute illness.

- Proper shoes are a must. Take more than one pair of comfortable, well-broken-in shoes. If your trip involves river rafting or beach time, get a pair of sandals that strap on in such a way that your feet will not come out of them when walking over rough or rocky ground.

- Avoid purchasing medicines in other countries. Take extra medications with you and carry them in their original containers, if possible. Carry copies of your prescriptions to avoid customs hassles.

- Be cautious about taking medicines for travelers' diarrhea, especially those available over-the-counter in other countries. Prepare for this by checking with your physician before you leave home. Travelers' diarrhea is a common problem. Be prepared to cope if it hits your grandchildren, too, and be aware that adult dosages may be dangerous for children. Discuss this with your physician.

Health Insurance Abroad for Grandparents

The insurance you have at home may not be honored in many countries. Bear in mind that traffic accidents are the leading cause of serious injury to American travelers in foreign lands. What about the possible need for blood transfusions where the supply is not up to U.S. standards and needles may be reused? Confirm your health insurance benefits before you leave home.

In such cases, the best solution may be immediate evacuation by air back to the United States. This is an enormously costly undertaking that can be offset by evacuation insurance. Be sure you read the fine print and understand whether you are getting the right protection in the right countries and that no unreasonable limits or requirements are involved.

Great Activities for Grandparents and Children

There is one thing you can say about today's grandparents: There is just no way to generalize about them. But if you are reading this book, the chances are good that you do not expect to spend your vacation with your grandchildren sitting in a rocking chair on the porch.

In fact, many of the activities that are suitable for parents and children are equally suitable for grandparents and children. But why not look for something a little different that will make the trip extra special? Naturally, your decisions will depend on the ages and abilities of your grandchildren as well as your stamina and theirs. Children have a shorter attention span, so don't take it personally if they do not want to spend the entire afternoon looking at your stamp collection. Think about how much you have to share, not just on this vacation, but also on the next and the next after that. Here are some ideas to help you:

- Share something you really love with your grandchildren. Maybe you have a special interest in art, music, or baseball. Maybe you sail or square-dance. Maybe you love Italian food. Show your grandchildren the best of it.

- Grandparents are the guardians of the family history. Take some time to tell your grandchildren family stories, and show them pictures that will help them understand and appreciate their personal history.

- Take your grandchildren to the place you (or their parents) grew up.

- Do something together that your grandchildren never do—go to the opera, the ballet, or the racetrack.

- Take your grandchildren shopping.

- Teach your grandchildren a new skill—quilting, woodcarving, fly-fishing—and spend some time working on improving that skill.

- Select a book that has some meaning for both of you and read it aloud over the course of the time you are together.

- Participate together in a charitable activity—serving a meal at a homeless shelter, doing a charity walkathon, or grocery shopping for someone in your community who is housebound.

One of the great pleasures of grandparenting is treating your grandchildren to things they might not otherwise experience. If you are thoughtful and realistic about your travel plans and expectations, try to be creative and generous, set guidelines and limits, and insist on fun and mutual respect, you will both have a vacation memory you will cherish forever.

Chapter 7
Today's Special-Needs Travelers

The introduction to this book listed a few of the more important benefits of travel. Happily, those benefits apply equally to people traveling alone or in company, with or without children. Surely they also apply to people who are challenged physically or otherwise—perhaps even more so.

In years past, Americans with special health needs or limitations rarely ventured beyond our shores—if they even left their homes. Today the world is becoming more willing and able to accommodate travelers with special needs. As a result, people with limited or no vision as well as those who require wheelchair access are enjoying travel as never before; even people who require sophisticated medical care (such as dialysis) can obtain it in many places throughout the developed world.

Little was done for physically challenged citizens of average means until the passage of the Americans with Disabilities Act (ADA) in 1990. This farsighted act mandated access for disabled persons to all public transportation, public facilities, and retail establishments within the United States. Indirectly, the act created a demand for accommodating such travelers overseas, but in many places, provisions for travelers with disabilities are still limited.

Before the end of the twentieth century, a blind man reached the summit of Mt. Everest under his own power, and another, aided only by his guide dog, hiked the longest backpack route in the nation, the Appalachian Trail. Another sightless person, this time a woman, climbed Mt. Kilimanjaro.

Think What You CAN Do, Not What You Can't Do

The point of this chapter is not to urge you to climb mountains. Rather it is to emphasize that no matter what your limitations and challenges may be, you can do what you want with your life by focusing your mind and energies on achieving specific goals.

The level of your determination is the most important factor in whether or how well you achieve your goals. In this respect, you are no different from people without disabilities.

Pursue your goals with spring-steel determination. Acquire all the training you can; practice new skills every way you can. Do this and you will find yourself living a far more exhilarating life than you may now believe possible.

Yes, some sightless persons climb mountains, others ski down them, and some backpack along wilderness trails. Wheelchair users rock climb, play basketball and tennis, and compete in marathons. Others routinely get themselves into vans and drive anywhere they want to go, including long-distance trips to participate in conferences and other events. Many who have lost limbs enjoy ski racing. One of the hardest-fought events of many marathons is the wheelchair competition.

Wonderfully inspiring as all these sports and recreational activities are, many challenged people prefer to concentrate on their careers. By so doing they make enormous contributions to the world. Blind—or otherwise handicapped—musicians, entrepreneurs, and inventors have enormously enriched our lives.

Traveling with Special Needs

Whatever our physical abilities, most of us quickly learn our way around our home and hometown. We accommodate our lives to the bumps in the sidewalk, the uneven stairs, and the narrow doorways. But many people still deny themselves the pleasure of travel to unfamiliar places, fearing that their physical limitations will restrict their access and enjoyment.

As building standards and government regulations more appropriately address "special needs," and the travel industry recognizes the importance of all travelers, options and resources expand exponentially. Hotels, tour operators, airlines, trains, and cruise companies throughout the world welcome travelers young and old whose lives include limiting conditions.

As you are planning your itinerary, here are some points to keep in mind:

- Talk with your physician. Your doctor may be able to provide you with names, resources, and travel tips, as well as important documentation (see below).

- Pack light. Plan a layered wardrobe of garments that are suitable for various occasions and temperatures.

- Carry your medications. Although it may increase the bulk of your carry-on, carry your medications in their original containers and do not take any chances on lost luggage. If your medication requires refrigeration, carry a small cooler or use the resources of the carrier or hotel.

- Get your documents in order. Be sure to pack written copies of all prescriptions. Carry copies of recent medical reports if you are in treatment or have a potentially recurring condition. If you use syringes or if you have implants that could set off metal detectors, carry a letter or certificate from your doctor.

- Inform your travel companions, including tour operators and airline or cruise personnel, of any medical conditions you may have, how to recognize symptoms, and where you keep medications. If you travel with a motorized wheelchair, a respirator, or a guide animal, be sure to discuss it at the time you book your travel.

- Stay on schedule. If you are crossing one or more time zones in your travels, make sure that you have planned your medication schedule according to your doctor's recommendations.

- Ask about available assistance. Air and cruise lines, tour operators, and hotels will provide wheelchairs and other forms of help if you ask in advance.

- If you are traveling with your own wheelchair, be sure the agent tags your chair as well as your suitcase at check-in. You may be able to take your own chair as far as the door of the plane. At that point, you will transfer to a boarding chair that can roll down the narrow aisles. Your chair should be sent below to the baggage compartment, but it is a good idea to remind the attendant that it is yours and should not go back to the terminal. Be prepared to remove or secure all loose items, such as footrests or cushions.

- Plan for your arrival. It is easy to get so caught up in the plans to get there that you forget to arrange for what will happen when you arrive.

- Know the mechanics. If you travel with medical equipment, be sure to take extra parts and tools in case you need to make a midtrip repair. Know how and where to get new batteries or supplies in your destination city. If a lighter-weight, narrower wheelchair is available, consider purchasing or renting it for your trip. Many travelers recommend a narrowing device to help squeeze the chair through aisles and doorways.

- Fight jet lag. Travel in off-peak daytime hours whenever possible. Get rest before you travel and avoid alcohol during your flight.

- Book ahead for comfort and safety. Although many hotels now have "handicap" rooms, they may be limited in number; off-season travel may give you a better chance at getting one.

- Ask for what you need. You know in advance what your needs are—elevator access, adequate door width, ramps, Braille signage, grab bars—so it makes sense to confirm as much as possible in advance. Do not expect hotel staff, transportation personnel, or people on the street to read your mind. If you need a hand, ask for it. All the better if you can ask in the local language!

- Confirm, reconfirm, and be flexible. A few days before you leave home, call and reconfirm the details of your transportation, special meals, and hotel accommodations. But remember that even the best-laid plans can go awry, so be prepared to enjoy the adventure, whatever it brings. In case things go very wrong, travel insurance can cover medical emergencies, canceled flights, or lost baggage.

- Vote with your wallet. If you have a choice between an airline or hotel that can provide for your needs and one that cannot, favor the former with your business and let them know why. If you discover that the accessibility is less than promised, share the information with your fellow travelers when you get home.

- Tap into the resources. Most up-to-date travel guidebooks offer information for travelers with impaired mobility on accommodations, air and train travel, auto rental, and hotels and restaurants. There are also Web sites, newsletters, and tours targeted to those with various abilities, and your local auto club or travel bookstore will also have numerous resources available. If you ask around, you might also find a travel agent who is knowledgeable about special-needs travel. One of the most comprehensive on-line resources is the Society for Accessible Travel and Hospitality at www.sath.org.

Traveling with Special-Needs Friends or Relatives

- Research the trip before committing to it. Be sure that the disabled person's needs—especially those that cannot be delayed—will be met as required at every stage of the journey.

- Two federal acts provide protection for those with special needs: the Air Carrier Access Act and the Americans with Disabilities Act.

- Investigate the route in detail as required by the needs of the person's abilities. When you are in unfamiliar places where you may not understand the local language, your ability to avoid or solve problems will be greatly reduced over what you could achieve at home.

- Avoid peak times when facilities are overcrowded. Not only will this make your trip less stressful and improve the quality of the service you obtain, it will also cost less.

- Discuss any special needs the disabled person has with every transportation company you plan to use. For best results do this several weeks in advance of your trip.

- Do not assume your companion wants help. People with limited vision or mobility may resent a guiding arm, and not everyone in a wheelchair wants a push.

If you have a specific condition, consider the following:

Diabetes

- To avoid delay in customs, carry a letter from your doctor describing your need for syringes.

- When traveling in a group, inform your group leader and teammates of your condition. Familiarize them with hypoglycemia, and instruct them about what they should do if hypoglycemia strikes.

- Before venturing into any non-English-speaking country, learn how to say "Sugar or orange juice, please; I have diabetes" in the local language.

- If you will cross multiple time zones, check with your health care provider about adjusting your insulin schedule. Avoid making large changes in your mealtimes without consulting your doctor.

- If you need to inject insulin when flying, bear in mind that insulin will enter the syringe more readily when you are aloft than at sea level.

Dialysis

Talk with your specialist about dialysis centers that are available in resorts, on cruise ships, and in cities worldwide. Internet sites for more information are listed in Appendix C.

Mobility Limitations

- Keep in mind that at any point during the trip the members of your party may be obliged to carry their luggage, and this could happen when you are pressed for time to make a connection. Plan how this will be done.

- Make sure you do not take more gear than can be carried. Plan carefully, simplify, and reduce your clothing as much as possible.

- If you will need a wheelchair at airports, request one when making your reservations. Find out whether you can request door-to-door assistance, and make sure someone will be available to assist you in claiming your luggage.

- Allow extra time so you will not miss your flight if you are waiting for a wheelchair.

- As you check in, repeat your request for assistance when you deplane.

- Do not accept short flight connections. If you will be changing planes in an unfamiliar airport, insist on at least two hours to make the plane change.

In today's unpredictable travel environment, your most valuable carry-on item is your sense of humor: It's weightless, guaranteed to improve your trip, and is sure to make you a welcome guest. Plan well, travel safely, and have fun!

Service Animals

Although the best-known service animals are guide dogs, other species are also employed, including small monkeys and cats. Service animals are not pets.

Under the Americans with Disabilities Act (ADA), privately owned businesses serving the public, such as restaurants, hotels, retail stores, taxicabs, theaters, concert halls, and sports facilities, are prohibited from discriminating against individuals with disabilities. The ADA requires these businesses to allow people with disabilities to bring their service animals into business premises in whatever areas customers are generally allowed.

The ADA defines a service animal as any animal individually trained to provide assistance to a person with a disability, regardless of whether the animal has been licensed or certified by a state or local government. To minimize difficulties with access for a service animal, equip the animal with an identifying cape, and, of course, keep it on a leash. Careful research can help you avoid problems, especially during international travel.

Significant quarantines may be imposed, particularly in Hawaii, Australia, New Zealand, and Great Britain. Investigate the requirements and restrictions for your destination with your travel consultant or embassy well before your departure date.

There are many resources available to people with special needs, and many of them include valuable information about travel. Every medical condition has Web sites, newsletters, and organizations devoted to the interests of individuals and families it affects. Some of them are listed in Appendix C. Your personal physician, travel medicine specialists, travel agents, and libraries can provide additional resources.

It is comforting to know that there are people who have circumstances similar to yours, and it is inspiring to see how they have met and triumphed over their difficulties. They and many others are working hard to remove the impediments to safe, convenient, and pleasurable travel. Whatever your abilities, travel can recharge your batteries and fill you with renewed creativity, stimulation, and awareness, so start planning today!

Part III

Travel Modes

Chapter 8
Commercial Transportation

When you travel by public conveyance, you entrust the health and safety of your family to the commercial operators of the service. In general you must accommodate yourself to the schedules and policies of the transportation company—something that is likely to be more challenging when you travel with children. As with all other aspects of your travel, careful preparation is imperative.

There are advantages to each form of travel. Consider your time, your budget, your trip goals, and, of course, your family as you choose one.

Train Travel

Parents planning a family vacation or a trip to see distant relatives may never even consider train travel. This is unfortunate because train travel is the closest thing to driving your own car.

Whether you are on a short excursion or an extended journey, there are many reasons to travel by train. Here are a few to consider before you book your next trip:

- Train travel is fun. As a train passenger, you can sightsee, converse, eat, stretch, walk, sleep, read, drink, play cards or other games, and daydream—all while you are on the way to your destination. Although a car passenger may be able to indulge in a few of those activities—albeit with less ease—the driver must maintain highway vigilance, especially in unfamiliar territory. This often means the driver misses out on many of the pleasures of travel and arrives at the destination exhausted.

- Train travel is popular. Train travel is becoming more popular, and many cities in the United States and abroad have excellent rail service.

- Train travel is economical. The costs of rental cars and gasoline in Europe and many other parts of the world are high compared to U.S. rates. Add insurance, value added tax (VAT), other taxes, and parking charges, and car travel may not look quite as attractive.

- Trains get you where you want to go. Because trains make efficient use of resources and are used by both commuters and tourists, they stop at communities large and small. For example, Europe's Eurail system reaches some 30,000 cities, towns, and villages.

- Train travel is comfortable. For space, convenience, and romantic ambience, trains win hands-down over plane, coach, and car.

- Train travel is flexible. Many travelers rent cars, thinking it is the only way to have the freedom to be spontaneous. However, with rail passes and frequent train departures, you can stop on a whim, explore, and reboard when you are ready.

- Train travel is convenient. If coach and car excursions from hotel to hotel have you packing and unpacking every day, consider the convenience of day excursions by train. Choose a central location, check into your hotel, and then take day or overnight train trips to explore the countryside. As a bonus, you will be traveling with the locals, who can share culture and conversation as you go. If you are planning extended stays in several distant locations, consider traveling by train between them, and then renting a car to explore the local scenery.

Whatever part of the world you are planning to visit, using trains will enhance your journey. Most rail passes can be purchased before you leave home, and many countries and rail services offer guidebooks (for example, *Europe by Eurail*) for travelers that are complete with maps and itineraries.

Checklist for Family Travel by Train

- Make reservations as far in advance as possible so that you can obtain the family seating you want.

- Traveling with an infant, luggage, a stroller, and a car restraint seat is easier if two adults are available to help.

- Carry a personal supply of essentials, such as toilet paper, soap, towels, blankets, or coats.

- Take along extra snacks.

- Take plenty of games and toys.

- Study your route in advance and make a game of following your progress on a map.

- Have your children make lists of the countries, states, cities, and towns you pass through.

- Every hour or so, take your child on a trip through the train for exercise.

- Ask about checked baggage. On some trains you will check most of your belongings and carry on only the supplies you will need for the trip.

Subways

A city's basic form of public transportation is much the same everywhere: It's cheap, crowded with locals, and frequent. This is true whether you are taking the subway in New York or Los Angeles, the BART in San Francisco, the Metro in Paris, the Tube in London, or the Vaporetto in Venice. The last is the fleet of large motorboats running routes along Venice's Grand Canal. Like subways elsewhere, the Vaporetto can be physically challenging for anyone caring for an infant. Unlike subways, the Vaporetto provides marvelous views.

Many subway systems are equipped with sturdy gates designed to prevent riders from boarding without paying. Often wheeled luggage will not go through in the normal way; you may have to pick it up and carry it or turn it sideways and drag it through. In some stations you may be able to get an attendant to open a gate for strollers, wheelchairs, and luggage access.

In many subway systems it can be hard to tell whether you are going in the right direction on the right track. The easiest way to be sure is to know the name of the final destination of the line you are using. A wall map of the system can be found in most stations and in many subway cars, and leaflets containing the same map in miniature may also be available.

Cruising with Kids

Many travelers find that cruising is the most relaxing and comfortable of vacations. Whether your entire vacation with the children is spent aboard ship or a cruise is just a sidelight, advance planning can make the experience more pleasant for everyone.

Day cruises designed for families are increasingly common in popular island and coastal destinations and offer great opportunities to test your family's seaworthiness before you commit to a week or more afloat.

Ask your travel agent and visit the Internet for family cruise information, either by destination or cruise line. Look for cruises that have special onboard activities and shore excursions for kids—if your children are old enough to go on such adventures without you. Bring your children into the decision-making process. Once you have narrowed your choices, ask for detailed information on:

- numbers and ages of children on the cruise

- numbers and qualifications of crew members who will be supervising children

- safety and security practices

- whether children's programs are available when you plan to travel

- what activities are planned for children both onboard and onshore, such as special meals or overnight programs

- whether baby-sitting services are available onboard

- whether cribs and playpens are available, if needed

Optional shore excursions offer visits to local attractions and provide greater security than wandering around on your own, but they substantially increase the cost of the cruise, so check ahead. You may be able to prebook shore excursions when you buy the cruise, or the cruise line may allow you to order them from your stateroom aboard ship.

Most cruises to the tropics offer a variety of water activities. A favorite with children, snorkeling is one of the safest of water activities when common sense precautions are observed. Consider investing in snorkels and masks that fit properly and, before you leave home, take your children to a pool and have them practice using their new snorkels before they try it in the ocean.

Here are some shipboard safety tips:

- In doorways of older ships, look out for raised ledges.

- If the lock on your cabin door requires use of a key from the inside, leave the key in the lock when you are in the cabin. In case of power failure or nighttime emergency, you do not want to have to hunt for your key or search for the keyhole.

- Use the ladder provided to enter and leave the upper berths.

- Never throw smoking materials (or anything else) overboard, even if you think they are extinguished.

- Ship stairs are different from ordinary stairs, and the decks may be damp from sea mist. Walk cautiously and use handrails. Wear rubber-soled (not crepe) shoes for extra traction on decks.

- On deck, a cool breeze can mask the effects of the sun. Use plenty of sunscreen or lotion, wear sunglasses, and limit your sun exposure.

- If you think you may be subject to motion sickness, check with your physician before your cruise and choose a cabin in the most stable area: amidships (middle section) on one of the lower decks. Medication is available to prevent this problem.

- You will be required to participate in a lifeboat drill. Be sure to cooperate in familiarizing yourself and your family with the procedure. Set a good example to your children by taking the drills seriously.

Cruise ship sanitation has vastly improved in recent years. Perfect scores of 100 percent are being awarded to many more vessels, thanks to vigilant efforts by the industry. Ships calling at U.S. ports are inspected and rated by the Centers for Disease Control (CDC) and are required to maintain detailed records of cleanliness, food preparation and storage, refrigeration, food temperature, water supply, and so on.

The ratings are available on the CDC's Web site, www.cdc.gov/nceh/vsp, where prospective passengers can quickly determine the performance of a ship they are considering. The ratings are based on a single inspection, so look at a rating history to get a better overview of the ship's performance.

Air Travel

Flying on scheduled commercial airliners is far safer than going the same distance by car. Yet far more people fear flying than driving. If this is a problem for anyone in your travel party, read the section on "Fear of Flying" in Chapter 3.

Although most airlines have removed all restrictions for traveling with newborns, many pediatricians recommend keeping infants away from crowds, especially during the first three months. Do everything possible to move away from people who are sick or coughing. Use common sense and consider the mother's health as well. There is no sense risking the health and safety of either mother or child.

If your child was a premature birth or has a medical condition, such as congenital heart disease or anemia, check with your pediatrician before traveling by air. If your child has a temperature or is irritable, crying, tugging at his or her ears, vomiting, or experiencing diarrhea, it seems sensible to postpone your vacation until the condition clears. No one will have a good time.

If you are flying with an infant, allow extra time at the departure terminal so you can board the plane with a baby who is warm, dry, well fed, and sleepy. If you are breast-feeding, a window seat may provide better privacy; you and your child are much safer remaining belted in your seat than going to the aircraft's lavatory for breast-feeding. For older children, a window or bulkhead seat may offer greater comfort and safety.

In general, try to book nonstop flights to minimize takeoffs and landings, which can inflict painful changes in cabin pressure.

The Federal Aviation Administration (FAA) does not require passengers to purchase separate seats for children under two years of age, and they prohibit the use of booster seats. They do recommend the following guidelines for child-restraint systems (CRS):

- children under 20 pounds should be restrained in an approved rear-facing CRS

- children weighing 20–40 pounds should use an approved forward-facing CRS

- children weighing over 40 pounds should use the standard lap belt that is attached to all airline seats

Ask your travel agent for the current child restraint requirements for your chosen mode of travel.

If you plan to take your child's car seat aboard a plane, make sure first that it is approved for airline use. Most car seats are not designed to work with airplane seat belts, and car seats that are airplane-compatible are considerably more expensive than those designed exclusively for cars. For additional information consult with the airline when making reservations or contact the FAA's consumer information line.

Besides coping with greater sensitivity to changes in cabin pressure, flying with an infant involves changing diapers, feeding, and keeping the baby content and quiet. The best traveling infants sleep through most of their flights. However, do not use medications to make little travelers drowsy for two reasons: (1) You should never give medications except for medical reasons; and (2) drowsiness-inducing pills often have the opposite effect. Instead of an infant who only wants to sleep, you may have one who only wants to fuss and scream.

Federal regulations do not allow flight attendants to handle soiled diapers, no matter how carefully wrapped—a sensible health measure. So at 30,000 feet you are on your own in coping with diaper changing. There are only a few options:

- Fly short hops so you can do the changing on the ground.

- Some new aircraft have changing stations in the lavatories; inquire before making reservations.

- Use three of the airline's blankets and your changing pad to convert the lavatory into a workable changing station.

- The worst solution is to use fold-down tray tables—your own and the one for the next seat. Usually this works only if someone in your party has that seat. If a stranger occupies it, he or she may object strenuously and be supported by other passengers seated nearby.

- Have a plastic bag handy to hold soiled diapers until you can dispose of them after deplaning.

A few passengers on any airliner are likely to have a cold, especially if you are traveling during the holiday season. The air inside the passenger cabin will be recirculated many times through filters that do not remove all of the contaminants, so you and your children may possibly be exposed to some viruses brought aboard by other travelers.

This poses a greater risk to toddlers than to infants. Cold viruses travel on particles of mucus and are more likely to be picked up from a contaminated surface than from the air. Toddlers tend to scramble over everything and put their fingers in their mouths. A well-wrapped infant can be kept from contact with possibly contaminated surfaces.

This puts the task of avoiding cold viruses on the parent. Be careful not to put your fingers near baby's mouth, nose, or eyes after you touch any surface—armrests, trays, and so on—that could be contaminated. Without being obsessive about it, wash your hands—and your toddler's—as often as you can while traveling. You can use antiseptic wipes or waterless washing solutions without leaving your seat.

Luggage

If your luggage exceeds the allowable weight, you may have to contend with this problem at every stage of your vacation. Your options are limited if you are faced with exorbitant charges to get your overweight or oversize gear aboard an aircraft about to fly from Budapest to Cairo. You can pay up, abandon the items in question, or take a later plane. This last choice may give you time to ship your overweight or oversize gear by lower-cost land transport—if you can locate such a company quickly. Be aware that while restrictions are easing throughout Europe, customs and airline regulations elsewhere in the world can range from bad to impossible for travelers on a tight schedule.

If you shop on the trip, have your purchases shipped home by the seller. This avoids adding your new treasures to the load you are already lugging along. If you do this, buy with a credit card so you have some recourse in case a merchant fails to ship your purchase.

Weight restrictions aside, if your group has more packages than all of you can carry yourselves, consider how you will cope where no porters are available and you are pressed for time to make connections.

Sightseeing by Bus

If you and your children book an organized tour overseas with a travel company, there is a good chance part of the journey will be made by bus.

Coach tour itineraries are of two kinds: (1) daily round-trips, where you board a bus in the morning and are returned to the same hotel that night; and (2) one-way trips, where the bus moves you and all of your luggage to the next destination on your itinerary. Some tour companies sensibly do not allow infants; those that do should be researched thoroughly. However, without inconvenience or extra expense, you can stay in the hotel with your infant on round-trips, but not on one-way trips. If any of the latter are involved, determine how long you will be confined to the bus between diaper-change stops. Beware of just checking the distance on a map—difficult terrain may result in very slow progress. Obtain all the information you can before committing to such a trip with an infant.

Whichever mode of travel you choose can be exciting and rewarding for you and your family, especially if you are prepared, healthy, and avoid injury.

Chapter 9
Travel by Car, SUV, or RV

Although the stress of kids whining and fighting in the backseat might seem inevitable on a long road trip, the pain is easily avoided—or vastly reduced—with good preparation. Instead of being an ordeal, taking your children on the road can lead you from one fun-filled experience to another and can be a priceless time of family togetherness.

When you are not hampered by luggage restrictions, you can load your vehicle with as many changes of clothing as you want. You can take a playpen, a stroller, and an almost unlimited supply of games and puzzles to keep the kids occupied. You can also pack along skis and snowboards, scuba gear, even a sailboard or two—whatever equipment you think you will use on the trip, and rent a small trailer if you need more space. Even though it is possible to ship everything by air or another form of transportation, keep in mind that each additional item adds hassle to your journey and may substantially increase your cost.

How Will You Get There? . . . and How Will You Get Around?

Before you jump in the car—or rush out to rent a motor home—you might want to take a closer look at your driving options and consider whether they fit your family's style and your trip.

The Family Car

Assuming that the family car is safe enough for your family at home, it has one great road advantage: familiarity. You know how it handles, you know its quirks, and you know where and how children can be strapped in safely. When you are navigating new territory, you should have your mind on the roads and scenery, not on figuring out how to handle an unfamiliar vehicle.

On the other hand, once you have assembled all the bikes and backpacks, suitcases and coolers, the family car may be too small for the road trip you have planned. Remember that this is a vacation, so try to avoid filling up the backseat with luggage and then stuffing the children in between. They will be miserable—and so will you. You may be able to haul some of that gear on top of the car or stow it in a small trailer, but be sure to go for a test drive prior to your trip to get comfortable with the car's altered handling. If you are planning to settle into a campground or hotel and take side trips from there, the family car may be a great choice.

Sport Utility Vehicles

You may already be driving an SUV as your family car, but if not, this larger vehicle might give you the space and comfort you need for your road trip. Remember that SUVs have a higher center of gravity, so they may be somewhat less stable in high winds and on fast curves. Like cars, sport utility vehicles now come in a variety of sizes, from one barely larger than a station wagon to huge luxury cruisers. If you select a heavier model, you will gain stability and safety, though you may sacrifice something in gas mileage. Many of today's SUVs come loaded with entertainment options to keep backseat riders busy, and they have plenty of room for larger families and ample gear. Plus, the higher chassis gives passengers a better view of passing scenery. If you drive a sports car or compact at home, allow some time before your trip to practice navigating and parking the much larger SUV.

Minivans

Minivans are usually well appointed for family travel. They often have a fold-down (or removable) third seat to allow for gear, plus they are easy to handle and park. Some minivans have backseat entertainment options. If you are renting a minivan, check the make and model's safety record, and be sure you know what's required to gain access to the spare tire.

Full-size Vans

Potentially an entertainment center on wheels, the full-size van is typically customized from a commercial vehicle designed for hauling substantial loads. They are usually strong and stable, but if you are considering a van as your vacation vehicle, be sure to test for comfort, visibility, and child safety first. Since they are designed for commercial use, some full-size vans may not offer the comfort you need for a long road trip. Does the van have enough seats and windows for family cruising? Will it fit in a standard parking spot or go through a car wash? A van can be outfitted with almost any kind of gear, including a raised roof, but if your route includes auto-ferry or train rides, check vehicle height restrictions ahead of time.

Motor Homes

Plenty of room for everybody and everything, a place to cook and sleep, and even a bathroom—what could be better? True, motor homes are appealing for those attributes and others, but there are a number of shortcomings you should consider as well. Motor homes can be difficult to steer, unstable, and very hard to handle in windy conditions. And even though they are loaded with entertainment options, the temptation for small passengers to wander around is great—and completely unsafe. Most motor homes are designed for the cruising comfort of the driver and one passenger but have less desirable options for the family members in "the back." Plus, when you reach your destination, your motor home will be cumbersome for any local exploring (especially off-road) and taking short jaunts to the grocery store.

Whatever kind of vehicle you decide upon, be sure to take it for a test drive, and check it over carefully before you set out and regularly along the way. Check tires and fluids, and make sure all seat belts are in good working condition and safe and suitable for your passengers. If you plan to rent a vehicle, make sure the rental company does not mark vehicles with telltale decals. You might even consider renting a vehicle with navigation equipment that will guide you to your hotel and other destinations.

Then fill the tank, buckle up, and happy trails!

The Advantages of Driving

There are many advantages to being your own driver on a vacation. Here are some of the big ones:

- You can haul far more gear than is practical for public travel. The only limit is how much your vehicle will safely carry. You can easily expand this by renting and towing a small trailer or installing a luggage box on the roof of the vehicle.

- Your travel schedule in a car is under your control at all times.

- Family travel by auto is usually less expensive and more convenient than by public conveyance.

- Its flexibility makes going by auto the preferred mode of travel with an infant.

Car-Travel Tips

- Agree in advance that frequent stops will be made, and schedule the trip accordingly. Families should not attempt to go as far between stops as adults routinely do.

- Before you start out, let your children run around for a while and tire themselves.

- Except when your children are sleeping, avoid driving more than two hours without giving your children a chance to get out of the car and run around for a few minutes. This will allow them to burn off the excess energy they would otherwise put into poking and teasing each other.

- Attempt cross-country travel by car with an infant or small child only when two adults can share the responsibilities of driving and child care.

- Take advantage of stops to stretch your own legs; you will be more alert and a safer driver or navigator.

- Bring liquids and snacks—a day's worth of supplies. Avoid sodas and sweets in favor of water, milk, diluted juices, crackers, cheese, and dried fruit.

- Get an adapter for your automobile's cigarette lighter socket to warm bottles and soups for your little one.

- Bring an ice chest (available in many sizes) to keep drinks cold.

- Provide for hot and cold climate needs.

- Make child restraints an unbreakable rule of the road.

- Test your safety-seating arrangements for your child well before you leave on your trip. Otherwise, you may have trip-delaying, last-minute problems.

- Make sure everyone's lap/shoulder belts are buckled—and stay buckled—whenever the car is moving. Do not start the motor until everyone is buckled up. You can turn this into a race or other game to make it more appealing to children.

- Air bags are a serious hazard to children riding in the front seat. Always seat kids in the back.

- Think ahead about sleep patterns, and organize your trip to minimize the disruption of your daily meal and sleep schedule.

- Bring a variety of toys, games, and music.

- Carry a cellular phone and roadside emergency phone numbers.

- Never leave children alone in a vehicle for any reason, anywhere, at any time of day or night, for any length of time, in any kind of weather.

- Request and expect appropriate conduct from your children when traveling in the car.

- If your destination will include a large gathering of people, let your children adjust to the group and respond to people at their own pace.

- Consider joining the Automobile Association of America (AAA). The AAA's invaluable maps, directories, discounts, and emergency road service make membership a highly attractive proposition.

Child Restraints

Auto crashes are a leading cause of death and injury to children in the United States. Laws in all fifty states require that children be provided with restraints suitable to their age, height, and weight, a simple safety measure that cuts fatalities and injuries to children by more than half. Specific requirements may vary, both in the United States and abroad; research the rules for your destination before leaving home.

The rear seat is the safest place in the vehicle for all children, especially those under twelve, to be secured. If a small child must ride in the front seat, move the seat as far back as possible and turn the passenger-side air bag off if the vehicle has a cutoff switch.

In general, four types of child restraints are available:

1. Infant car bed, for low-birth-weight infants including preemies. Follow the instructions in the vehicle owner's manual and make sure the bed is secured so that the child's head is toward the center of the vehicle.

2. Rear-facing infant restraint, for infants from birth to twenty pounds. Some models can be used for children up to thirty pounds.

3. Forward-facing child restraint, for children one to four years of age who weigh twenty to forty pounds and are 26 to 40 inches tall.

4. Booster seat, for children four to eight years of age. The booster seat adapts the car's standard seat belts for safe use by children weighing

between forty and eighty pounds. This seat should be used until the child can be secured safely in adult safety belts, usually when the child is about 4 feet and 9 inches in height.

Always test restraints and always use all buckles in the restraint. Also, be sure you are being a good model for your children. If you do not use your seat belts and enforce seat belt rules every time you get in the car, you cannot expect your children to become safe passengers.

Marvelous Miles and Joyful Jaunts

Kiddie boredom is an enemy that must be locked out if a long trip with children is to be an enjoyable experience for everyone in the car. The answer is to keep plenty of things handy that will keep them happily occupied.

Plan for games the whole family can play. Alternate between private time and family time. In private time, your children draw, write postcards to their friends, listen to their own music on earphones, keep a journal, or play games by themselves until they tire of it.

When that happens, you will know the moment is right to declare family time, when everybody joins in a sing-along or some other group activity, such as having each person tell part of a story, which is then continued by the next parent or child.

Plan for at least twice as many activities as you think your family can cram into the trip. Discuss some of these activities with your children before the trip to make sure they are prepared and willing, but keep a few surprises in store. Many books packed with suitable games and puzzles are available; some of them are listed in Appendix C.

Between private time, family time, snack time, rest-stop run-around time, and gawk-at-something-unusual-going-by time, the day will fly, and your family will bond ever closer as a result of spending this time enjoying each other.

Packing for a Land Trip

The great appeal of loading up the family vehicle and taking off on a vacation is that you can take everything you could possibly want. You can, but should you?

Too much gear can create a tremendous hassle every time you stop for the night. Unless you are superbly organized, your essentials for a night on the road will likely be buried under piles of things you will not need until you get to your destination. Here are some tips to help you:

- Pack what you will need on the road in small duffel bags. Load these bags last, so they will be on top. Duffels are available in many sizes and colors, so you can even color-code your baggage, for example, by person, activity, or day.

- Avoid overloading the car to the point where the occupants are too crowded for comfort.

- Be sure the driver's rear visibility is not impaired by baggage.

- Consider renting a small trailer to provide more space.

Driver Beware

Any parent knows that even a sleeping child in the back seat adds an element of distraction to the driver's responsibilities. Those occasional loving glances at your small passenger take your mind off the road for a few seconds. And what if you are carrying a child who is wide awake—or more than one child? For each added distraction, your focus—and your road safety—is reduced.

This means that today's drivers, with or without children, are more distracted than ever and more vulnerable to accidents caused by their momentary loss of focus. Consider these very common in-car hazards:

- Fussy or fighting children. Much as you love them, your kids demand atten-tion. The best solution is early prevention: Plan for plenty of games, music, snacks, and blankets to keep your youngsters occupied and comfortable, and set (and enforce) rules for passengers. For example, your rules might include: no throwing, no poking, and no screaming. Just as important as seat belts, common-sense rules can give you a measure of control when you need it most. Regular stop-and-stretch breaks allow children to burn off excess energy outside of rather than inside the car. If your child is fussy, pull over and take some time to deal with the problem before resuming your travels. Always allow extra travel time when your children are in the car.

- Pets. Your children are held securely in place with seat belts, but the family dog may be bounding between seats, licking your face, or leaning across your chest to stick its head out the window.

- Cell phones. A huge asset when you are late, lost, or in need of assis-tance, nonetheless cell phones—both handheld and hands-free—cut into concentration. The attention you give to the phone conversation is atten-tion removed from the road. Not only are you more likely to miss signals and signs, but your response time is slowed for the unexpected hazards of traffic.

- Entertainment. Although tapes, CDs, and DVDs may provide a welcome distraction for passengers, they often demand entertainment management from the driver. The time you spend looking for the disk or the song you want, or glancing at the screen, is time your eyes are off the road.

- Technology. The wonders of modern technology can help you navigate unfamiliar roads, make last-minute reservations, collect your e-mail, and conduct business meetings on the road. But each of these options demands your concentration and some require additional dexterity for handling keypads, clickers, or voice commands.

- Food. Whether it is the first double latte of the day, a quick lunch on the run, or a full meal spread out on the seat beside you, food takes your hands off the wheel and your eyes off the road. Plus, with the added hazards of spills and choking, eating on the go is less a pleasure and more of a danger.

- Reading and writing. How many times have you glanced into a car and seen the driver studying a map, newspaper, magazine, report, or even a book? Reading and writing (including phone numbers and directions) should be reserved for times when the engine is turned off.

- Other distractions. Today's multitasking adults seem to think that they can carry their skills right into the car. It is not unusual to see people shaving, applying makeup, styling their hair, changing clothes, dressing children, or reaching around behind or beneath the seat for something they have dropped.

These distractions are often compounded—children plus food, cell phones, and writing—and their danger is often amplified by road conditions—darkness, rain, construction, or heavy traffic. The National Highway Traffic Safety Administration estimates that distractions play a role in 20 to 30 percent of all automobile crashes each year. You may think that you are saving time by doing something besides "just driving," but when that something else puts your family's safety at risk, is it really worth it?

Chapter 10
The Family Outdoors

In addition to adventure, fun, and togetherness, a camping trip or outdoor adventure can build your family's appreciation for nature and increase personal resourcefulness. Camping is usually more affordable than other accommodations, and it offers a great option for extended family and multiple family gatherings.

As with every other form of travel, preparation can make the difference between a camping triumph and a camping catastrophe. Planning, packing the right equipment, and preparing yourself for hazards can smooth the way to a great trip.

The Family That Adventures Together . . .

Although some people prefer packaged family-activity destinations such as Disney World, increasing numbers of people are setting their sights on greater adventure—mountain climbing, biking, rafting, sailing—and locations off the beaten track.

Like any travel experience, adventure vacations benefit from advance planning. If you are considering something "different" for your next trip, here are a few tips:

- Build your skills at home. If you expect to cover some ground on a hiking vacation, hike some easy trails near home to get in shape. If you will be spending time on the water, invest in swimming and water safety lessons before your trip. (More on water safety later in this chapter.)

- Road test equipment before you leave. Whether it's hiking shoes, skis, mask and snorkel, or baby carrier, make sure it fits properly and comfortably and does the job you expect it to do. Do not wait to discover problems when you are 3 miles into your hike.

- Consider everyone's abilities. Plan a variety of activities on your vacation so that everyone will have a chance to be challenged as well as to excel. Do not let the strongest/fastest or the weakest/slowest always set the pace.

- Involve your children in the planning. Books, magazines, television, and movies are full of information about your destination and can enrich your experience, especially if you share them.

- You don't have to go far to have fun. A trek in Australia's outback might be fantastic, but there are also wonderful parks, mountain ranges, lakes, oceans, or islands much closer to home to explore.

- Take advantage of abundant resources. There are scores of Internet sites devoted to family adventure travel. Start with tour operators, outfitters, and destinations and look for their family-oriented programs. Many outfitters have in-store travel consultants who can help you. And don't forget to talk with your friends who have traveled with their children.

Pre-trip Boot Camp

Take your family out to the local park and set up your tent and sleeping arrangements. Check out everything. Little things that are easily corrected in town can be a serious time waster or annoyance if discovered in the field. Make sure you and your children know how everything works.

This is the time to instruct everyone on how to recognize the poisonous trio—poison ivy, poison oak, and poison sumac. Ask your pediatrician for this information.

This is also the time to decide what you will leave behind and what you really need and will use. Having too much gear wastes time and energy you and your family could spend enjoying the trip.

What to Take for Safety and Comfort

Although a complete discussion of camping skills and considerations is beyond the scope of this book, there are six major requirements for having a happy camping experience with your children:

1. **Keep them warm.** Children lose body heat more quickly than adults do. A very small child might not be able to articulate discomfort, so parents should check skin temperature periodically to see if the child's skin feels cold. Dress children in layers so they can quickly adjust to changing conditions, and train them to put the clothing they take off into their backpacks so the items will not be lost. Long underwear can double as pajamas.

   A great deal of body heat is lost through the scalp, and a knit cap will do more to keep your child warm than almost any other garment. Mittens give greater warmth than gloves. Keep mittens from disappearing by attaching them to opposite ends of a piece of yarn that runs up one sleeve and down the other.

Mufflers and scarves are fine for adults, but they can be hazardous during rough play. Turtleneck shirts and jackets with hoods protect the neck in all but the bitterest cold.

2. **Keep them dry.** Clothing that allows air to circulate but keeps out the rain is best. A child who has been playing in the rain or snow is likely to have wet feet, so bring along plenty of extra socks.

3. **Keep them fed.** It takes more organization to provide unspoiled food and safe water on a camping trip than it does at home. Plan ahead so you can prepare one meal at a time. Outdoor activities generate great hunger, so bring along lots of healthy snacks. If possible, cut food at home and package in small snack bags for easy handling. (See more on picnics later in this chapter.)

4. **Keep them from getting lost in the wilds.** Most teenagers can take care of themselves with little supervision. And the tiniest kids can be kept on a leash—literally. But the ones in between are of the greatest concern. They are intensely curious, likely to be excited if the camping trip is an unusual experience for them, and capable of wandering off in an instant.

    Equip any child who may wander off alone with a cellular phone if it will work in the camping area. If not, give him or her a walkie-talkie (including backup batteries). Walkie-talkies have a range of up to 2 miles unless blocked by mountains. Also supply the child with a survival kit.

5. **Keep them away from dangerous animals.** Your pre-trip research may reveal whether dangerous animals share the area you want to camp in and hike through. Be sure to check with rangers or other local authorities regarding dangerous fauna. (More about animal hazards later in this chapter.)

6. **Keep them away from poison ivy and examine them for ticks that could carry disease.** This involves awareness, insect repellent, and, if you will be in brush or forest, long pants, long sleeves, and sturdy boots.

See Appendix C for additional resources on family camping.

Getting Ready to Hit the Trail

Here is a checklist to speed your preparations for your next camping trip. If you are ready for the small mishaps that result in cuts and bruises, you and your family will have a more enjoyable adventure. Enrolling the family in a first-aid class is a smart way to prepare for your trip, and you may want to look into other work-shops that will improve your experience, such as compass use, outdoor cooking, and so forth.

Camping First-aid Kit

You can purchase ready-made first-aid kits, but building your own is more eco-nomical. A complete list of items to put in your kit is included in Chapter 4. You may want to bring along your entire first-aid kit or assemble a kit specifically for camping trips. Select the items carefully, make sure they are protected from dirt and moisture, and after your trip be sure to restock any items you used.

Flashlights

The important thing about flashlights is to make sure that you have one handy at the moment you need it. The size and number of flashlights you carry will depend on the size and number of family members you have. Plus, you will want lanterns for tables and tents and a sturdy light source for your car. Headlamps may be more costly than handheld flashlights but they offer hands-free convenience. Children's lightweight flashlights are available with an automatic shutoff feature, and some small flashlights come with neck cords, which can prevent loss and ensure that the light is where you need it when you need it. However, beware of choking hazards.

Once you have decided on your flashlights, stock up on extra batteries. And take the time to talk about flashlight etiquette—no lights shone in the eyes, for example.

Bedding

Here's what you'll need for a comfortable night on the ground:

- tent and ground tarp
- sleeping bags
- Therm-a-Rest pads, cots, air mattresses, or foam pads
- pillows, stuffed in a trash bag or a large duffel bag
- comforters or extra sleeping bags if the weather is cool

Backpacks

If you and, most importantly, your smallest child, are not experienced in the outdoors, avoid taking any hike that will last longer than an hour. Each child who is
old enough should have his or her own water-bottle carrier and a small pack containing whichever of the following items they are old enough to use:

- a small first-aid kit

- sunglasses

- snack items such as trail mix and dried fruit

- toilet paper, just in case

- whistle to summon help

- watch

- compass

- small mirror (can be metal) for daytime signaling

- small flashlight

- walkie-talkie, cell phone, or both

- thermal blanket

- 20 feet of ⅛-inch braided nylon (Children should be taught how to tie it
  between two trees and lean branches against the line to make a wind-
  break.)

- bottle of safe water

- folding knife

- small notebook and pen

Other Gear

Here is some other gear that will make your camping trip easier:

- binoculars

- cooler

- camp stove and lantern with fuel for each, plus matches in a sealed
  container

- cooking and eating utensils

- safe water

- food

- clean-up supplies

- large trash bags (These have many uses, from hauling garbage to packing wet gear, so take extras.)

- old blankets for picnics, play spaces, and sundry other uses

- plenty of old towels for mopping up wet tables and many other camp chores

- maps, guides, and books or charts to help you identify local flora and fauna

- activity equipment, such as climbing or fishing gear

The Campsite

Here are some suggestions to make your home away from home more pleasant:

- Arrive early, otherwise you get your pick of the campsites no one else wanted—if any are still available. Selecting a site in the dark can be hazardous.

- Choose a campsite carefully to ensure the cooking area is away from brush, overhanging trees, and other fire hazards.

- In areas where flash floods may be a hazard, select a campsite on higher ground. Consider how rainwater will flow, and dig a small trench to guide the water around your tent.

- Arrange tents so that there are obvious pathways or "camp streets" to help people avoid tripping over tent poles and other hazards in the dark.

- Check your flashlights and batteries well in advance so that you do not find yourself at a remote location with very little or no light source.

- Rehearse the route to the rest rooms several times and establish rules about who can go alone and who cannot.

Campfires and Tools

Besides providing warmth, sitting around the campfire and gazing into its endlessly fascinating flames is one of the special joys of camping. It is a great time for singing, storytelling, and all sorts of family bonding.

Because of the danger of forest fires and for the protection of fragile ecosystems, there may be strictly enforced rules against campfires. *Build fires only in designated and approved sites, contain them carefully, and never leave a fire unattended—or a child unattended near a fire!*

If fires are allowed, you will probably have to supply your own firewood, although you may be able to buy reasonably priced dry wood near your destination. Green, freshly cut wood can be extremely difficult to ignite and miserably smoky once it's lit. Even getting dry wood to burn can be a difficult task for the inexperienced and unprepared camper. In addition to dry wood, you will need kindling and matches.

Always be sure to cover your campfire with sand or dirt before leaving the campground—*even if the fire appears to be completely out!*

On the Use of Sharp Implements

Axes. These long-handled cutting tools are swung over one's head and brought down with great force. A miss can be catastrophic because the ax head stands a good chance of winding up deep in your foot. At most public campsites, cutting down a tree is a crime.

Knives and hatchets. Cuts from camping knives and other sharp implements are common. Many people believe that dull knives and hatchets are safer than sharp ones, although the contrary is true. Sharp tools do the job faster, work with less force, and are less likely to bounce off whatever you are trying to cut. Practice using knives or hatchets before leaving home to gain some skill with them. When chopping wood, wear something to protect your eyes from flying chips: A wounded eye is a serious matter anywhere, but especially in the wild. Always wear boots or shoes while chopping wood.

Pets and Camping

The best advice is: Do not even think about taking pets along unless you have more than a year of family camping experience. Your children pose enough of a challenge out in the woods.

Even after you become old hands at camping, if you and your children love your pets, leave them at home, with a friend, or at a kennel when you camp. Your pets live in an artificial world and lead a cozy life where food comes in a bowl at regular times. As a result, their survival skills do not measure up to those of wild animals.

More reasons for leaving Spot at home include:

- Cats and dogs attract ticks and bring them back to you. In Lyme disease country, taking pets along increases your family's risk of becoming infected with this serious ailment.

- Pet food attracts animals and insects.

- Pets can easily become contaminated with urushiol resin by scampering through poison oak or poison ivy. The poison will stick to their fur and then contaminate you and your children.

- Even if your dog does not provide a meal for a coyote or a mountain lion, it may encounter a skunk or a porcupine.

- Your dog may fight with dogs belonging to other campers or howl in the night in the strange environment.

- And what do you do if your pet gets lost? You will get little assistance from park rangers or other campers. It will be up to you to find your pet.

No one needs these problems on a camping trip.

Picnics on the Go or in Camp

When you are on the road—near home or far away—picnics are a great option for family meals. In addition to fresh air and scenery, picnics can be a welcome relief from the physical restraints of car travel and other touring activities. But if you plan to dine alfresco, make sure your meal is safe to eat. Here are a few tips:

- Wash hands. When you are on the go, hand washing may be easy to over-look, but hands can easily contaminate food, leading to gastrointestinal problems. Waterless washing products are now widely available, so add them to your picnic basket, along with paper towels.

- Time it right. When you are traveling you can assemble picnics with pre-pared foods from restaurants. Keep hot and cold foods separate and eat the hot food as soon as possible.

- Use a cooler. Make sure the top fits securely and use about a quarter of the space for ice or cold packs.

- Keep the cooler closed as much as possible. Opening the cooler not only affects the temperature within but may also introduce contamination from dirty hands.

- Wash fruits and vegetables thoroughly. This may require some creativity when you are traveling, so take advantage of rest stops to give everything (and everyone) a good scrubbing.

- Keep meats tightly wrapped. Air and dirt can speed spoilage, so keep meats wrapped until it is time to cook or eat them.

- Cook meat and eggs completely. "No pink" is a useful rule of thumb for beef. Eggs should be cooked until firm.

- Use paper plates one time only. Food can become contaminated when plates are reused, so paper is preferable. Carry plenty of extras. Also carry trash bags so you can take your trash with you if no trash bins are convenient.

- Plan and prepare one meal at a time. Leftovers and food that is prepared far in advance are more likely to spoil, so limit your picnic preparations to one meal.

- Carry water and other beverages. Do not use lake or stream water for drinking or washing. Few water sources are entirely free of contaminants and many present significant hazards. There are numerous products on the market that claim to purify water, but the best way to purify water is to bring it to a rolling boil for at least a minute at sea level. Increase boiling time at higher altitudes.

- Lock up your food and remove your trash.

Wild Animal Awareness

The idea of seeing animals in the wild may be one of the attractions of the great outdoors, and depending on the animal, it may be one of the rewards. A doe and fawn grazing near your campsite, an owl hooting in a tree overhead, or a mountain goat making its surefooted way up a slope can be a thrilling encounter. On the other hand, a camp visit by bears, skunks, or snakes could be upsetting and dangerous for everyone concerned.

Here are some precautions you can take if you are confronted by any dangerous animals:

- Make sure your children can be depended on to not harass or approach any animal, whether it is a snake, rodent, or some larger creature.

- Be smart about food. Many wild animals, from mice to bears, are habituated to human food and know where to find it. Campsites might as well have flashing neon signs that say FREE FOOD HERE! Every morsel of food in your campsite—from pan scrapings to packed coolers to snacks tucked away in fanny packs—is a fragrant lure to wild creatures that could pose a hazard to you and your family. Before you set out, establish a careful routine for cleaning up and storing food, either by locking it in your vehicle or suspending it high overhead. Make sure that trash—wrappings, paper plates, empty drink containers—is deposited with equal care in appropriate containers with secure lids. Make sure that small children understand that food must be removed from pockets and packs and stowed securely before going to bed.

- Prepare yourself mentally to face animals that seem dangerous. Retreat slowly. Do not run from a predator, because running marks you as prey and encourages the animal to attack.

- If large predators frequent your destination, provide yourself with a legal weapon: pepper spray (if allowed) or a heavy walking stick or club.

- Keep your group together when in the wilds. A child alone is extremely vulnerable; a child within a few feet of an adult is comparatively safe.

- Make sure your kids do not confuse wild animals with the patient creatures found in petting zoos. Any wild animal that can be petted is almost certainly sick, very possibly with rabies, which is prevalent among wild animals in all of the contiguous forty-eight states.

Mountain Lions

Mountain lions are also called cougars, panthers, and pumas. Adult males can weigh up to 150 pounds and be 8 feet long from nose to tip of tail. Mountain lions are found throughout much of California, in other states of the Southwest, and even in Florida's Everglades. Increasingly, these magnificent federally protected great cats are adapting to urban and semi-urban areas, although they generally avoid confrontation with humans. Anywhere you hike while camping is likely to be mountain lion territory, so keep the following in mind:

- Keep children close to you and within your sight at all times.

- Finish your meal and wash your hands before setting out on a hike.

- If you see a mountain lion, do not approach it or try to corner the animal. Always make sure it has a clear way to escape.

- Never run from a lion. Running is what the animal's prey does, and it may stimulate a mountain lion's instinct to chase. Instead, stand and face the animal. Make eye contact. If you have small children with you, pick them up if possible so they don't panic and run. Although it may be awkward, pick them up without bending over or turning away from the mountain lion.

- Do not crouch down or bend over. A human standing up is just not the right shape for a cat's prey.

- Do everything you can to appear larger. Raise your arms. Open your jacket, wave your hat or anything you are carrying. Wave your arms slowly and speak firmly in a loud voice. Remain standing, face the animal, and throw stones, branches, or whatever you can reach without crouching or turning your back. Convince the mountain lion that you are not prey and that you are dangerous.

- In the unlikely event that you are attacked, fight back using pepper spray, rocks, sticks, or anything you can to fend off a mountain lion.

Large Grazing Animals

Most wild animals are too elusive for hikers to catch even a glimpse of them. Although bison, elk, moose, and other grazing animals will not think your tyke is food, they are dangerous if approached.

Bear cubs must be avoided even if Mother Bear is nowhere to be seen. You can be sure of two things: She is not far away, and she will attack if you get near one of her cubs. And stay clear of other young animals for the same reasons.

Above all, make clear to your children that animals in the wild are not the genial cartoon characters they love to watch or the tame and carefully selected creatures in petting zoos. Wild animals follow the law of the jungle; when in their territory, humans must pay attention to jungle law, or pay whatever penalty is imposed.

Dangerous Vacation Sports

When we go on vacation, we are tempted to engage in sports with which we are unfamiliar. This is to be expected and we must take every measure to ensure our safety. All sports have some degree of danger, but in some the "thrill factor" makes danger a necessary ingredient.

If you or your family members will be skiing, snowboarding, bungee jumping, skydiving, parasailing, scuba diving, hot-air ballooning, hang gliding, or operating motorcycles, all-terrain vehicles, snowmobiles, or jet skis, exercise great caution.

- Always inspect equipment carefully. Look for worn parts, damaged connections, and obvious signs of poor maintenance.

- Observe the operator in action. Ask to see company certifications and operator's licenses, and make sure they are current and cover the people who are actually operating the equipment or giving instruction.

- Ask what kind of safety training the operator or instructor has received.

- Ask about safety procedures and accident track record.

- You may get more candid information about the operator from unrelated sources—local sports stores, tour operators, or other hotels—so ask around.

- Find out in advance whether there are any restrictions on the sport and whether it is covered by your insurance policy or the operator's. Insurance may not cover death or injury from these sports. Check before you play.

- Take lessons. Follow all instructions exactly, and if anything is unclear, ask for additional guidance. Proper training not only reduces the likelihood of injury, but also lowers your liability if you or your child injures someone else while participating in the sport.

- Be aware that your teenage children may be eager to "get going" and may not be paying careful attention to instructions.

- If any protective equipment is available, such as helmets, goggles, or gloves, use it.

- Avoid these activities if you have had bone surgery of any kind.

- Make sure that your child is old enough, big enough, and mature enough to participate in the sport, and never let children under six "ride along" or be towed by any sort of motorized equipment.

- Before you participate in any sort of rough or impact sports, have a physical exam that includes informing the physician of what is planned.

Television and movies make these and other sports look effortless and exciting. It is tempting to think that we can just "jump on and go." But in dangerous sports, participation and competition can be fatal, especially with teenagers, who tend to take more risks than younger children. Plan carefully, exercise caution, and have fun.

Water Safety

Drowning is one of the leading causes of death of young children. Swimming and water play are so common in everyday life that we can forget how dangerous even a small amount of water can be to children. Water activities are a common feature of family travel, and the need for parental vigilance is paramount, wherever you are.

Because of pollution, disease, and the presence of dangerous wildlife (such as jellyfish and fire coral) it may not be advisable to swim or dive in rivers, lakes, or oceans in certain parts of the world. Check with the CDC and your travel physician for advice specific to your destination.

Young Children from Birth to Twelve Years

A very young child's head may be the heaviest part of the body, and unattended children can drown in bathtubs, buckets, coolers, toilets, and other places containing a surprisingly small amount of water. Never leave a child unattended in or near water. Regardless of their age, children around water must be watched by a designated adult at all times. Children can learn to swim at six months, but even a child who has demonstrated competence as a swimmer should not be left alone in the water. Even good swimmers drown.

Rafts, inner tubes, and "floaties" do not prevent drowning. A young child left alone in the water is at risk even if he or she is wearing a floatation device.

In addition to the hazards of drowning, extreme water temperature—both hot and cold—can be dangerous. If in doubt, do not put the child in the water.

Older Children from Twelve to Eighteen Years

Older children, even those who are skilled swimmers, are at risk in ponds, rivers, lakes, oceans, and even pools, especially when they overestimate their swimming abilities. In addition, the hazards of currents, entanglement, exhaustion, cramps, and panic can be compounded by the use of drugs or alcohol, with fatal results. Never swim alone.

Older children may be given responsibility to baby-sit or supervise younger children around water. Before they are allowed to do so, they should be trained in water safety and able to demonstrate appropriate lifesaving skills. Teenagers can be easily distracted, particularly by members of their peer group, and may be tempted to show off or otherwise be diverted from their responsibility.

Pools

The most popular place for water recreation and sports and probably the most common site for drowning is the swimming pool. Here are some basic rules for the pool:

- Never run near the edge.
- Never be in the water alone.
- Never be in the water during electrical storms.
- Never dive without the permission of the adult in charge.

- Never push or hold anyone under water.

- Never allow electrical appliances, toys, bicycles, tricycles, wagons, skateboards, or other hazards close to the pool.

- Always have a telephone poolside for emergencies.

- Every five-year-old child should learn how to swim.

- Always personally accompany a child five years old or younger into the water and do not leave him or her alone.

- A 5-foot high fence with a safety gate should surround all pools.

- Remember that swimming lessons and floatation devices are no substitute for supervision or observation.

Diving

Diving can be divided into two basic categories: surface and underwater. The latter includes snorkeling and scuba (Self-Contained Underwater Breathing Apparatus) diving. Both require swim fins and other equipment as well as training by experts. Pre-vacation pool practice is both sensible and fun.

If you or your children will be spending much time snorkeling or scuba diving, you may want to purchase masks before you leave home. A properly fitted mask sits comfortably on the face, does not leak, and can even be outfitted with corrective lenses. Rental equipment should always be checked carefully for leaks, scratches, tears, sand, and cleanliness. Always check with lifeguards or other local experts regarding water conditions and underwater hazards before swimming, snorkeling, or diving into unfamiliar waters.

Surface diving into pools, lakes, rivers, and oceans can cause head, spinal, and other serious injuries. The depth of the water must be determined before making the dive. In an emergency, when the depth cannot be determined, a feet-first jump should be done, but even then, serious injury can occur because of shallow depth or underwater hazards.

Never dive from bridges, barges, piers, or docks where submerged abutments, pilings, or discarded fishing line or hooks may be present but unseen.

Aboveground pools are too shallow for any diving and should be drained after every use. Since there is no fence around them, they are a great temptation for children and a serious drowning hazard.

Diving boards are found by older pools, but because of the risk of injury and the serious liability, many home owners have removed them. Resort and hotel pools may have diving boards, but no one—especially children—should use them without training, even the low ones.

Water Sports

In addition to swimming and diving, other water sports include sailing, motorboating, canoeing, kayaking, surfing, waterskiing, sailboarding, and jet skiing. All of them require a life jacket, except possibly surfing. All of them provide exercise and health benefits, but they can present some hazards, too.

Sailing has its own ancient code of safety involving the rules of the seas and safety on deck and while underway. Make sure that children are aware of the rules from the person in charge.

A canoe or kayak can be a very tricky boat to handle because it is so light. Some special instruction is necessary, particularly for young people.

Motorboats can be divided into two kinds: large and small. Adults operate the former, some with a crew. It is wise to ask that the person in charge explain the safety rules to your child. That way, the child is helped in avoiding injury and the parents can take note of the level of experience, care, and communication ability of the owner, captain, or crew.

Small boats are often operated by very young people who are not skilled in their handling, so parents should determine the boater's skill level before allowing a child to get in the boat. The child's own age, experience, and skill should be considered as well, and life jackets must be worn at all times.

Life jackets are very important in saving lives, so make sure that they fit properly and remain in place. It is tempting for youngsters to loosen or remove their life jackets because they find the jackets unattractive, bulky, or hot. Air mattresses, pool toys, inner tubes, water wings, and other floating toys are not safety devices and are no substitute for life jackets.

Sunburn

The need for sun protection is emphasized throughout this book, but water sports of all kinds expose children and adults to extremes of sun exposure. See the section on "Sunburn" in Chapter 3 for more information.

Many vacation destinations feature water activities such as swimming pools, water parks, and water slides. Appropriate instruction, swimming lessons, and safety awareness are critical to protect a child's health in and around the water. Proper training can overcome fear, build confidence, and increase enjoyment of the water's many pleasurable pastimes.

Appendix A
Dr. Coleman's Prescription for Safe Baby-sitting

Baby-sitters and Nannies—Guidelines for Parents

If you have an infant, more than a decade and a half will pass before you are free of the frequent or at least occasional need for a competent baby-sitter. Peace of mind while traveling without your children, or even while just out for the evening, begins with having a reliable person looking out for your children. Ideally that person would be a loving grandparent, sibling, or other responsible adult. Realistically it will probably be a neighborhood teenager, or someone found through classified ads or by calling an employment agency. Avoid frantic last-minute searches for a baby-sitter by developing a stable of dependable, mature baby-sitters you can be sure will take good care of your infant or children.

The worst place to cut expenses is on what you pay baby-sitters. However, just paying more does not necessarily guarantee that your baby-sitter will be a safe person to leave your baby with. If you live in California, you can get help with this question by calling TrustLine; otherwise, call Child Care Aware (see below).

The use of professional nannies is growing daily. A person who is hired to clean or cook has many responsibilities; watching a child should not be one of them. Phone everyone who has given an applicant a written recommendation. People who wrote a glowing recommendation to ease their own misgivings about firing a nanny may reveal the cause in a friendly phone call. Also, ask for a written resume, even if it is brief. Pay particular attention to unexplained gaps in the applicant's work record, which may indicate problems he or she does not want to reveal. If the nanny is associated with a baby-sitting service, ask about insurance coverage.

In addition to checking on the applicant's work record, ask the following questions:

1. What activities do you like to participate in with children?

2. Have you had to deal with an emergency while watching children?

3. Have you been certified recently in infant/child CPR and first aid?

4. What will you do if my child cries all day?

5. How will you respond if my child says, 'You are not my Mom and I don't have to do what you tell me.'?

6. What would you do if my children started fighting with each other?

7. What if my child refuses to eat or take a nap?

8. What will you do if you are not feeling well?

9. If you were away from the house and an accident occurred, what would you do?

10. Do you drive, or do you have access to a car in case of emergency?

11. Why do you enjoy working with children?

Trust your instinct. Even if a nanny arrives with a personal referral and years of experience, it does not guarantee she will have good chemistry with your family.

Child Care Aware

Child Care Aware (800–424–2246) is a national referral program that helps parents locate licensed day care providers. It may be able to supply names of day care services in towns on your itinerary.

TrustLine

TrustLine
California Child Care Resource and Referral Network
111 New Montgomery
San Francisco, CA 94105
(415) 882–0234 or (800) 822–8490

A state agency in California's Department of Social Services, TrustLine was organized to tighten California's system for monitoring at-home child care providers. For a fee, California parents can have a potential child care giver screened for criminal convictions and substantiated child-abuse allegations. The record search only covers California, but for an additional $24, the FBI will search nationwide.

There are two weak spots in the system: (1) Applicants who pay the fee to qualify themselves are allowed to submit fingerprints by mail. If they have some-thing to conceal, it is a simple matter to substitute a crime-free friend's fingerprints for their own. If you pay the application fee, ink the applicant's fingers yourself. (2) TrustLine has no way of checking whether foreign-born applicants have criminal records in their country of origin.

More than 32,000 at-home caregivers have cleared the TrustLine background check and are currently registered on the agency's database. Each year about 7 percent of applicants are refused registration because of criminal backgrounds, such as convictions for murder, manslaughter, sexual assault, and willful child cruelty.

You may find other trustworthy caregivers through religious organizations, visitor and convention bureaus, hotels, and other resources such as especially trusted friends.

Additional Baby-sitter Tips

Your baby-sitter may have a lot more experience with children than you do—or a lot less. Be sure that you have covered all the bases before you walk out the door. A little extra effort will ensure your child's safety, the baby-sitter's peace of mind, and an enjoyable respite for you. Consider the following suggestions:

- Treat your baby-sitter with respect. A good baby-sitter is worth his or her weight in gold, so take time to discuss expectations and arrangements in advance. You may even want to set up an introductory visit to familiarize the sitter with the kids and house and to talk about details. As you are rushing out the door is not the time to start this conversation. Be sure to talk about hourly pay, transportation arrangements (to and from your home), special activities, and emergency information.

- Remember that things that are routine for you may be novel or even frightening for a baby-sitter. If your child requires special medical attention, food preparation, or bedtime rituals, be sure to explain each activity carefully. If your child has "just a little diarrhea," an unprepared baby-sitter could be alarmed. Advance warning will allow the sitter to prepare and deal with the problem. Also, do not just assume that your baby-sitter will be willing to deal with anything contagious (flu, mumps, head lice), so be sure to ask first.

- Spell out your house rules very carefully. Which phone, television, and foods are off limits? Do you want the sitter to answer the phone? Discuss bedtimes, TV times, and computer rules. If you have pets, be sure to talk about their needs and behavior as well. Explain your philosophies clearly regarding eating habits, crying, and discipline, and ask the sitter to explain hers as well.

- Be sure your sitter can handle the job. If you have more than one child or if you will be away for a particularly long time, an inexperienced baby-sitter may find the job overwhelming. One solution is to allow the sitter to recruit a trusted friend to help. Some parents pay both sitters; others expect the two to split the hourly rate. In either case, discuss these arrangements in advance.

- Prepare the kitchen. If you expect your baby-sitter to feed your children, make sure there is plenty of food available. Discuss meal preparation and cleanup, and be sure to explain where meals are—and are not—to be eaten. A few snacks (sodas, fruit, chips) for the sitter are always welcome.

- Try to stick to the schedule. Sure, you're looking forward to a "free" evening, and sure, it is easy to lose track of time if you are having fun. But give your baby-sitter a realistic guess at your return time and talk about what you will do if you are going to be late. Do not assume that late is all right; your sitter may have other commitments.

- Allow your baby-sitter the courtesy you would extend to any businessperson. Your doctor may see you at a moment's notice in an emergency, but do not expect him or her to be happy if every visit is an emergency. The same goes for your sitter. Plan far in advance for really big events, within a week or ten days for normal weekend sitting: If a last-minute situation arises, your sitter is more likely to be responsive if you have treated her with respect on other occasions. If you have to cancel, do so as early as possible.

- Talk about household changes. If you are lucky enough to have a regular baby-sitter, take a moment occasionally to talk about what's new. If you have a new doorbell, dishwasher, or dog, be sure to mention it. If your normally cheerful child is having a tough time with teething, bring it up.

A great baby-sitter is a trusted companion for your children and a friend to your home and family. The foundation you establish at the beginning of your relationship will pay off in the months—or years—ahead. Take a little extra time now, and be sure to let your sitter know that you welcome questions and are prepared to help her or him meet the challenges of the job at hand.

Guidelines to Set for Baby-sitters

Parents should review this material and make sure they leave a safe house in which the baby-sitter can safely care for their children. It is the parents' duty to childproof their home, and it is unreasonable to expect a baby-sitter to provide a higher level of child care than parents themselves give their children.

In more than twenty-five years as a pediatrician, the following are the most common and problematic issues I have observed about baby-sitters:

- They are too casual and too young to watch an active child or children.

- They are not trained in CPR.

- They are visiting on the phone instead of watching the baby.

- They have visitors while baby-sitting.

- They are not aware of dangers to children of various ages, especially at playgrounds, in backyards, and around water, even in kitchens and bathtubs.

Once parents are sure the home is as child-safe as possible, they should review these guidelines with the baby-sitter:

1. In an emergency, do not panic but act fast. Concentrate on what needs to be done, then do it.

2. If there is a fire or smoke, get the children out of the house first. Do not try to fight the fire. Do not stop for anything until the children are safely outdoors. Take the children to a neighbor and call 911, the Fire Department. Then call the parents.

3. In the event of illness or accident, if it is an emergency, call 911.

Make Baby's Every Environment Safe

The Kitchen

If you can, make the kitchen off limits for toddlers and babies. If this is not possible, be extra-alert when they are in the kitchen, especially when cooking is going on. Make sure curious children are never permitted to go in the kitchen unless an adult is there.

Young children are curious; they want to explore and try new things. This natural urge is what motivates them to master skills and learn, but it can also put them in harm's way. Do your part to encourage a child's sense of adventure and at the same time help him or her avoid injuries. Be alert to what a child in your care is doing every minute, and be quick to check on the child if he or she is suddenly very quiet; this is often a signal that the child is into some mischief.

- Stove. Be alert to prevent children from pulling scalding hot pots down on themselves. Watch that the child does not turn on the knobs or touch hot pans. Turn pot handles inward so the child cannot reach them. Keep matches in a place too high for little people to reach.

- Appliances. Keep the cords wound up and out of the child's reach.

- Household chemicals. Be sure that all household chemicals are properly stored. Thoroughly clean all spills to prevent slipping.

- Plastic bags are not toys. A child can suffocate with a plastic bag over his or her head.

The Bedroom

Watch for common poisons such as cosmetics or medications. Store handbags that may contain sharp objects, small coins, medicines, or cosmetics. Be careful of jewelry boxes, scissors, and other potential dangers.

The Bathroom

Check with parents regarding bathroom habits. Young children should not be left alone in the bathroom. If the child requires privacy, leave the door open slightly and never leave the child alone in the tub. Always check to see that the medicine cabinet is locked and all razors, blades, medications, cleansers, or other potential hazards have been properly stored out of reach before allowing the child into the bathroom. Make it clear to the child that the toilet is not a place to play. Reinforce good bathroom hygiene.

Stairways

Make sure that safety gates are fastened securely at the top and bottom of the stairway. When carrying a baby up or down stairs, hold onto the handrail. Check to see that the basement door is locked.

The Living Room

Remove fragile or potentially hazardous items. Watch out for crawlers and toddlers pulling on lamp and telephone cords or probing electrical outlets.

Outdoors

Do not let children play in the street. Do not let the child play in the garage or with any sharp or large garden tools. Keep the child away from outside machinery such as air conditioners and lawnmowers. And never take your eyes off children around water. Be especially alert when a child is in a wading pool, at the beach, or near a lake. A potentially life-threatening emergency can arise quickly.

Tips for the Baby-sitter

Keep doors locked and do not open them to strangers. Never leave the children alone in the house. Stay awake. Do not have friends over to visit. Stay off the phone except for emergencies.

When discussing the baby-sitting assignment, agree on what food, if any, will be provided for your consumption. Pick up after yourself.

If you are like many young adults, baby-sitting may be your first employment experience. When you baby-sit, you are in business for yourself and the parents are your clients. Baby-sitting is an opportunity to hone your people skills; what you learn in coping with your client family will be invaluable in your later career. Here are some basic ideas for your consideration:

- Try to work for people you know.

- If the clients are new, get referrals from neighbors or friends.

- Agree in advance on the number of children to be cared for.

- Make sure the parents know that they are obligated to return at the agreed time.

- If you have school during the week, you may want to set limits on your time.

- Establish a clear understanding of your duties with the client. If you are expected to do housework in addition to caring for and supervising children, insist on additional compensation.

- Baby-sitting can be a win-win arrangement: The parents need a reliable babysitter; you need to make some extra money. Make sure that you are treated fairly or refuse the assignment.

- Set up a transportation plan to and from the job.

- Obtain the following information from the parents:
  - their cell phone number
  - location of, and phone number for, where the parents will be
  - phone number for local police, fire, doctor, and poison center
  - phone numbers for responsible relatives or friends nearby, if possible
  - any special instructions, such as medication, feeding, and so on
  - rules regarding bedtime, TV, snacks, and so forth

Fact sheet for this date/these dates only: _____

Where we will be: _____

Phone: _____

Will return by:_____

Special instructions: _____

_____

_____

Meals (wash your hands before handling food!):

Give no food except _____ at _____

_____ at _____

Medication needed: _____

_____

_____

_____

Sleep (when, clothes, blankets, window, heat, etc.): _____

_____

_____

_____

Bath: at _____. DO NOT LEAVE CHILD ALONE IN BATH.

Play (where are toys, books, clothes? Avoid stove, hot water, stairs, sharp objects, medicine, machines, open windows, electricity, street, animals, matches): _____

_____

Other instructions:

1. Keep outside doors locked (from inside only), and do not open to strangers.

2. The only people to be admitted in our absence are: _____

_____

Do not let anyone else in! Tell him or her to come back when we are home.

3. Keep phone lines open for important calls.

4. I expect the following deliveries and calls. Here's what to do: _____

_____

Use the back of this sheet for messages or information for us.

- Have the parents show you where you can find:
  - cups, plates, or other eating utensils you may need
  - cleanup supplies in the event of a spill
  - diapers, clothing, bedding, and food
  - electricity and gas shutoff stations (in the event of an emergency)
  - fire extinguishers and fire exits
  - thermostats
  - first-aid supplies
  - flashlights

Baby-sitter Information Sheet

The longer you plan to leave your children with a baby-sitter, the more detailed your instructions for that person should be. How smoothly things will go in your absence depends greatly on the completeness and clarity of your written instructions. If you set up your baby-sitter information sheet on a computer, it will be easy to change and add information as necessary and then print copies for each occasion.

If you have more than one child, you may want to make up a separate sheet of instructions for each child or provide space for each child's needs on the master sheet. If you have a child that requires special care, include as many details as necessary, even if this means adding a second sheet. A sample information sheet will look something like the sheet at left.

Appendix B
Plan a Successful Return Before You Leave

If you just flew back from the Caribbean, your mind may still be at the beach, to the detriment of your productivity and, possibly, your job security. To derive the maximum benefit from your trip with the minimum disruption to your earning power, plan in advance how you will get up to speed when you return to work.

Are You Ready to Leave the Office?

Vacation plans often involve a series of lists: things to do, things to buy, things to pack. While we are focused on what to take along, it is easy to lose sight of what we are leaving behind and what that could mean when we return home.

If you are an experienced traveler, household preparations become routine: arranging for the care of pets and plants, notifying neighbors, canceling the newspaper, and so on. But have you made equally thoughtful arrangements for your workplace? Here are a few things you may want to consider before you run out the door:

- How will calls be handled? It may be appropriate to leave a voice-mail message explaining that you are unavailable until a specific date and who to contact in case of emergency. But if you work out of your home, such a message may compromise the security of your vacant residence. Is there someone who can temporarily answer your phone or pick up your messages? Forwarding your calls to someone else may be more satisfactory to your customers and can often be accomplished through the phone company. Be sure you leave clear instructions on what to tell callers. Do you want them to know that you are unavailable? Out of town? On your honeymoon? On vacation?

  And what about e-mail? It may be tempting to plan on picking up your personal e-mail at an Internet café when you finally arrive in the Seychelles. But can all work-related messages be treated as casually?

Again, you may want to have your electronic mail forwarded to someone who can respond immediately and give you (or someone you designate) a heads-up on critical matters.

- Who are you likely to need to call about work-related matters? If you can get through your trip without calling home, it will be more of a true vacation. But if you must call in, it is a good idea to decide ahead of time who your personal and business contacts will be and let them know that you might be calling. It is also a good idea to make a note on your phone list about time differences, so you will not inadvertently call in the middle of the night.

- Who is responsible to cover the bases while you're gone? Rather than turning over your entire workload to someone else, consider parceling out time-sensitive tasks to several people. Be sure that everyone knows who to go to if there is a serious problem.

- Make contact before and after. Your clients and professional colleagues will appreciate a courtesy notice before you leave, especially if it means a very important project will be left in limbo while you are away. (Everybody's pet project is very important—at least to them.)

- Don't forget to call and say hello when you return. Most of us lose track of other people's vacation schedules. A friendly call creates goodwill and sets the wheels back in motion.

Before you leave, make a start-up list for your return—a list you may want to take with you on vacation. (You can always throw the paper away if it tenses you up.) When you have had a really relaxing vacation, you may find that toward the end of your trip you start to grow anxious about the work awaiting you at home. Or perhaps your stress level is so low that you spend weeks trying to reestablish your rhythm at the office. You can ease both symptoms before you leave home by making a list of work in progress, including who is handling what while you are gone, and your commitments, including all critical dates and deadlines falling within the first two weeks of your return. Make your list descriptive and thorough, but not so complicated that you will not review it when you are divinely relaxed.

On your first day back at the office, prime yourself to answer questions about your vacation with something like, "Had a great time. I'll tell you all about it after work." You will be busy enough without giving hourly travelogues to your curious coworkers. Schedule a busy first day packed with challenging activities. This will get you off to a fast start at making the first month after your return—rested physically and refreshed mentally and emotionally—your most productive period of the year.

Protecting Your Home While You Are Away

Minimize the problems you will encounter when you return by first ensuring that your home will be safe while you are away. Any time your home is unoccupied—even if for only a few hours—it becomes an attractive target for burglars. That's the reality. However, the perception burglars get when they cruise your neighborhood looking for an unoccupied house is what counts. Here are some ways to make your home look occupied:

- Do not advertise your absence with signs such as newspapers and throwaway flyers littering your driveway, trash cans left out, or an accumulation of mail spilling out of the box. Other strong indications that a home has been vacant for several days or weeks are unmowed lawns, unraked leaves, uncleared snow, and lights left burning all day.

- When leaving home for more than a day, arrange for a reliable person to pick up papers and otherwise keep the front of your house looking like it is occupied. Often neighbors will be happy to do this for you, with the understanding that you will do the same for them when they take a trip.

- If you will be away for a week or longer, stop all deliveries, including newspapers and mail.

- Two or three people are always home somewhere on your street. Find out who they are and get on good terms with them. Ask them to keep an eye on your place when you are away and call you or the police if they spot any suspicious activity at your home.

- Set up timers for lights to come on and off during evening hours so your home looks occupied.

- Arrange for any necessary maintenance, and for the payment of utility bills, while you are away.

- Choose a responsible person to care for any pets, children, aged family members, or plants you leave behind.

Organizing a Healthy Return

Your trip is not done until you have appropriately treated any sickness you may have acquired while traveling.

1. Even in the absence of any symptoms, after departure from a malaria-infested area, continue antimalarial treatment for the time specified by the

medication (which can vary). Most antimalarial medication is taken from one to four weeks after arriving home. Severe illness accompanied by high fever may develop weeks, months, or even years after you return from an area where malaria is endemic. If this happens, tell your doctor to consider the possibility of malaria. Physicians may not be familiar with the clinical signs of malaria if they practice where malaria does not exist, so you must alert them. If you have traveled to malaria-endemic regions, advise the medical personnel that you could possibly be infected with malaria before donating blood.

2. If a returning traveler has diarrhea—or any change in normal bowel functions that persists or worsens in spite of treatment—a thorough diagnostic workup is required. See your doctor promptly. Changes in diet, hepatitis, drug-resistant bacterial infections, or intestinal parasites may be responsible.

Travelers to both heavily populated and remote areas sometimes return home with uncommon illnesses. They may notice nonspecific symptoms, such as muscle aches or headaches. Next they typically experience gastrointestinal or respiratory problems, urinary discomfort, high temperature, or jaundice. As soon as you feel that you may have acquired an illness in your travels, see your doctor, who may refer you to a travel medicine specialist.

If we are a bit sluggish the first few days after a vacation, we tend to blame it on the speed of today's jet travel. That may be true, especially if you have flown east through several time zones, as when returning to the United States from Asia. Most of us experience milder jet lag when we fly west. Allow yourself a little time to adjust.

Questions Your Doctor Will Ask If You or Your Child Comes Back Sick

If you return from a trip and have nonspecific symptoms or fall ill, see your physician immediately to prevent a serious illness from developing. Be ready to answer the following questions:

1. What immunizations did you receive before your trip?

2. What preventive measures did you take prior to traveling to areas where malaria is prevalent?

3. Where did you travel?

4. How long was your stay?

5. What did you eat, drink, and do?

6. What diseases do you believe were prevalent in the area(s) you visited, such as malaria, cholera, or schistosomiasis?

7. Were you around anyone who was sick?

8. Were you sick at all during your trip?

9. How long after returning home did your symptoms begin?

10. Is anyone else with whom you traveled sick?

11. Is anybody at home sick who did not travel with you?

After investing tremendous time and energy in your preparations and travels, it is not uncommon to feel a little let down. So it would be a good idea not only to plan your wonderful vacation, but also to plan something special for you upon your return, for example, a movie or dinner out. Although it may be the last thing on your mind, this is also the best time to update all of your checklists and notes so that they will be ready to travel the next time you are. (The longer you put this off, the more likely you are to forget the things you promised yourself you would remember to add to your list!)

Here are a few suggestions to think about for quality renewal time close to home:

• Spend time with special friends or family; they enrich your life.

• Keep active and fit by enjoying your favorite exercise or sport.

• Remember that you have wonderful things to visit close to home, such as art museums, an arboretum, or simply window shopping.

• Attend a special event: Check the entertainment section of your newspaper. You may even develop a new interest after seeing something new.

• Spend time at a retreat. Plan a weekend away by treating yourself to a deluxe hotel weekend with breakfast in bed.

The world is full of opportunities for renewing the spirit and filling your life with the joy of living. When you plan your time for relaxation, remember to leave the "guilties" at home. You will always have time to take care of the things you have left undone. The key to healthy travel is careful planning and taking charge of details, because peace of mind is your best traveling companion.

Appendix C
Recommended Resources

Books

In addition to the books that are listed here, there are many helpful and beautiful books on travel that address almost every subject and destination imaginable. Always look for the most current edition and verify information before you leave home. Facilities, conditions, and restrictions can change quickly.

American Academy of Pediatrics. *Red Book 2000*. Report of the Committee on Infectious Diseases. Elk Grove Village, Ill.: AAP. This book is an encyclopedia of pediatric infectious diseases and is especially helpful to the medical professional.

American Automobile Association. *Traveling with Your Pet. The AAA Pet Book.* Orlando, Fla.: AAA Publishing, 2002. This indispensable guidebook lists "more than ten thousand pet-friendly, AAA-rated lodgings in the United States and Canada."

Auerbach, Paul S., M.D. *Medicine for the Outdoors*. Guilford, Conn.: The Lyons Press, 1999. This book offers helpful information on outdoor travel, especially in wilderness areas.

Backer, Howard D., M.D. *Wilderness First Aid. Emergency Care for Remote Locations.* Hones & Bartlett Publishers, 1998. The National Safety Council and the Wilderness Medical Society have collaborated to put together this comprehensive manual.

Bezruchka, Stephen, M.D. *The Pocket Doctor: A Passport to Healthy Travel*, 3rd edition. Seattle: The Mountaineers, 1999. This is a valuable resource for common travel problems.

Bittenbinder, J. J., and William Neal. *Tough Target: The Street-Smart Guide to Staying Safe*. Philadelphia: Running Press, 1997. This book offers a hard-on-crime approach to personal safety.

Bree, Loris and Marlin. *Kids Travel Fun Books*. St. Paul, Minn.: Marlor Press, 2002. This is an easy-to-carry resource for making traveling more fun.

Brown, Duane. *Flying Without Fear*. Emoryville, Calif.: New Harbinger Publishing, 1996. This is a good resource for those afraid to fly.

Bundren, Mary Rogers. *Travel Wise with Children: 101 Educational Travel Tips for Families*. Edmond, Okla.: Imprint Publishing, Inc., 1998. This relatively small book is packed with outstanding ideas on how to keep children educated and entertained.

Cardone, Laurel. *How to Pack: Experts Share Their Secrets*. New York: Fodors, 1997. This book discusses everything you need to know about packing, from how to buy luggage to how to pack for your return trip.

Cure, Karen, and Mark Sullivan. *Travel Fit & Healthy*. New York: Fodors, 2001. This is an excellent source of information if you want to begin an exercise regimen or continue yours on the road.

Dupont, Herbert L., M.D., and Robert Steffen, M.D. *Textbook of Travel Medicine and Health*. St. Louis, Mo.: B.C. Decker, Inc., 2001. This is a thorough textbook for health professionals.

Hanson, Eric, and Jeanne Hanson. *The Everything Kids Travel Activity Book*. Holbrook, Mass.: Adams Media Corp., 2002. This book is an excellent source for entertainment and activities for the traveling child.

Harrold, Glenn. *Overcome the Fear of Flying*. Divinity Publishing, 2002. This book will help you get over your fears.

Johns Hopkins Children's Center. *First Aid for Children Fast*. Batavia, Ill.: DK Publishing, 1995. This book is clear and simple, with instructions and outstanding pictures for first-aid needs.

Lansky, Vicki. *Baby Proofing Basics—How to Keep Your Child Safe.* Minnetonka, Minn.: Book Peddlers, 2002. This book provides simple and practical safety tips and guidelines for choosing products and equipment for children.

Lansky, Vicki. *Dear Baby Sitter Handbook. A Handy Guide for Your Child's Sitter.* Minnetonka, Minn,: Book Peddlers, 2001. This is a clearly written guide for baby-sitters and for those who must choose them.

Lutz, Eric. *On the Go with Baby, A Stress-free Guide to Getting Across Town or Around the World.* Naperville, Ill.: Sourcebooks, Inc., 2002. This very practical book focuses on baby-oriented situations involving travel.

McAlpin, Anne. *Travel Tips You Can Trust.* Orlando, Fla.: AAA Publishing, 2002. This is a very fundamental and useful book for all travelers.

O'Brien, Tim. *The Amusement Park Guide: Coast to Coast Thrills.* Guilford, Conn.: Globe Pequot Press, 2001. This book is valuable for the local as well as the long-distance traveler.

Perrin, Wendy. *Secrets Every Smart Traveler Should Know.* New York: Fodors, 1997. In each of the eight chapters of this outstanding book, Wendy Perrin includes a section on "where to find additional help." It should be a part of every traveler's library.

Pollard, Andrew J., and David R. Murdoch. *Travel Medicine.* Santa Fe, N. Mex.: Health Press, 2001. This "fast facts" book is excellent for its charts and tables and is particularly useful for travel in the United Kingdom.

Rose, Stuart, M.D. *International Travel Health Guide.* Northampton, Mass.: Travel Medicine, Inc., 2001. This lucid, comprehensive book is especially for the health professional and others interested in travel medicine.

Shapiro, Michael. *Internet Travel Planner: How to Plan Trips and Save Money On-line.* Guilford, Conn.: Globe Pequot Press, 2002. This book is invaluable for quick trip planning, and you can keep in touch on your laptop.

Smith, Robert P., and Stephen D. Sears. *Blackwell's Primary Care Essentials: Travel Medicine.* Malden, Mass.: Blackwell Science, Inc., 2002. This compact book should be in the library of every physician who advises people about travel medicine. It provides a synopsis of travel-related illness.

Spira, Alan M., M.D. *Common Sense First Aid for Travel and Home.* Beverly Hills: AMS Publications, 2000. This book is easy to carry and is filled with useful information.

Spurlock, Virginia Smith. *Traveling with Your Grandkids.* Orlando, Fla.: AAA Publishing, 2001. This one-of-a-kind book deals with a subject that is gaining increasing attention from the travel industry.

"Still Missing." Videotape & Resource Guide, New Day Films, 22D Hollywood Avenue, Hohokus, New Jersey 07423; (201) 652–6590. This is a serious study of childhood abductions.

Thompson, Richard F., M.D. *Travel and Routine Immunizations: A Practical Guide for the Medical Officer.* Milwaukee: Shoreland Medical Marketing, Inc., 2001. Although this book is intended for the medical professional, it may also be helpful for the sophisticated traveler.

Weiss, Eric A., M.D. *Wilderness 911, A Step-By-Step Guide for Medical Emergencies and Improvised Care in the Backcountry.* Seattle: The Mountaineers, 1998. The subtitle describes this book completely.

Wilson-Howarth, Dr. Jane, and Dr. Matthew Ellis. *Your Child's Health Abroad: A Manual for Traveling Parents.* Bradt Publications, distributed by Globe Pequot Press (Guilford, Conn.): 1998. The authors are very experienced in practicing medicine in Asia and tropical countries. They speak with understandable authority.

Zuckerman, Jane N., ed. *Principles and Practice of Travel Medicine.* New York: John Wiley & Sons, 2001. This medical textbook for health professionals emphasizes the prevention of disease for travelers worldwide.

On-line Resources

New Web sites appear and old ones vanish every day. By the time you read this, some of these sites may be gone. Use a good search engine to explore topics of interest, but be aware that many (if not most) sites related to travel have something to sell and many are based on one person's opinion. Do not rely on just one source for information about destinations.

Bargain travel

www.BiddingForTravel.com
"Our primary goal is to promote informed bidding when using priceline.com for your travel plans."

Camping and outdoor activities

www.nps.gov
National Park Service Web site

reservations.nps.gov
The National Park Service's on-line reservation site

gorp.com/index.adp
A commercial site with extensive information on outdoor activities

www.mountainzone.com
A mountain activities site

Car travel

www.nhtsa.dot.gov/people/injury/childps
Provides information on child safety in automobiles, including a chart for proper safety seat fitting

www.cdc.gov/ncipc/duip/spotlite/chldseat.htm
The CDC's pages on child passenger safety

Children's health

www.aap.org
The American Academy of Pediatrics Web site

Cruising

www.cdc.gov/nceh/vsp/default.htm

Customs, U.S.

www.customs.ustreas.gov/travel/travel.htm

Dialysis

www.globaldialysis.com
Offers connections to 10,245 dialysis centers in 115 countries

www.renalweb.com
"Links to Dialysis and Nephrology Resource Sites" lists dozens of Web sites and also offers a section on travel information.

Disabilities

www.afb.org
The American Foundation for the Blind Web site

www.agbell.org
The Alexander Graham Bell Association for the Deaf and Hard of Hearing Web site

www.dpi.org
Disabled Peoples International's goal is the full participation of disabled people in the mainstream of life, particularly those in developing countries.

www.wmedia.com
WeMedia Inc. is the leading media company covering issues most important to the millions of people with disabilities interested in a quality life without compromise.

Disease prevention

www.cdc.gov
The Centers for Disease Control and Prevention site includes information about diseases, including current outbreaks, vaccines, and treatments, as well as abundant information on health safety.

English-speaking doctors, finding them

www.istm.org
The International Society of Travel Medicine (ISTM) is the world's largest organization of professionals dedicated to the advancement of travel medicine, with more than 1,200 members in more than fifty countries.

www.highwaytohealth.com
This Web site has health information about the countries you select. If you carry a laptop on your trip, you may be able to access a map showing where the nearest English-speaking doctor can be found in the foreign city where you need medical care.

www.internationalsos.com
International SOS offers a worldwide network of clinics providing special services to travelers.

www.sentex.net/~iamat
The Web site for the International Association for Medical Assistance to Travelers

Evacuation insurance (See Trip insurance)

Fear of flying
www.AirSafe.com
Provides information on airlines and general flight safety, plus a page dedicated to resources for the fearful flyer

www.FearofFlying.com
Offers help from SOAR, Inc.

Federal government
www.dot.gov
Department of Transportation

www.faa.gov
Federal Aviation Administration

www.pueblo.gsa.gov/links/th6links.htm
Federal Consumer Information Center

www.tsa.dot.gov
Transportation Security Administration

www.state.gov
Department of State travel advisories and bulletins of interest to travelers

www.cdc.gov/nceh/vsp/default.htm
Vessel sanitation reports

www.aphis.usda.gov/travel/
U.S. Department of Agriculture site includes information on transporting animals and agricultural products

Heimlich maneuver
www.heimlichinstitute.org/howtodo.html

International health and travel
www.who.int/ith/
World Health Organization's informative site

Maps
www.Britannica.com
www.Globeexplorer.com
www.MapQuest.com
www.mapsonus.com
www.NationalGeographic.com/mapmachine/index.html

MedicAlert
www.medicalert.org
A subscription system that provides detailed medical information to health care providers all over the world. Anyone with severe allergies, medical conditions, or medications that could cause interactions, should consider this service.

Medical evacuation insurance (See Trip insurance)

Passports
travel.state.gov/passport_services.html
The Department of State passport information page

travel.state.gov/specialreq.html
Details the documentation required for children under fourteen

Service animal capes
www.nucapes.com—(215) 677–1352
www.wolfpacks.com—(541) 482–7669

Special needs travel
www.sath.org
The Society for Accessible Travel and Hospitality

www.accessible-travel.com
Books of interest to people with special needs

Theme parks

www.ThemeParkInsider.com

An independent source of information about theme parks, including discussions of safety

Trains

www.amtrak.com

View train schedules, search special offers, and book travel by train.

www.eurail.com

Everything you need to know about traveling through Europe by rail

www.thetrain.com

Plan your journey by train to the Grand Canyon.

www.viarail.ca/en_index.html

Rail travel in Canada

Travel information, general

www.medscout.com/travel_medicine

Provides extensive links to travel resources

Traveling with children

www.babies.com

This site is specific to rental equipment for babies. They claim all products are cleaned, well maintained, and approved by the Juvenile Product Manufacturer's Association. Items include cribs, strollers, pack 'n' plays, infant seats, beach toys, and more.

www.familytravelforum.com/index.html

www.familytravelguides.com

www.littleluggage.com

This company rents baby equipment to visitors to San Francisco and Los Angeles. All items are safety checked and sanitized prior to rental. Items include high chairs, cribs, strollers, and more.

www.rent4baby.com

This company rents baby equipment and stork signs exclusively in the Portland, Oregon, area.

Trip insurance

www.insuremytrip.com

Provides information on travel insurance policies from many different companies so travelers can shop for the best rates and coverage

www.travelguard.com

Insures more than four million travelers each year, protecting them against cancellation penalties, travel interruptions and delays, emergency medical expenses, lost baggage, and more

Trouble spot avoidance

www.travel.state.gov/travel_warnings.html

The U.S. Department of State's information is quite detailed and often gives warnings about specific regions and cities.

Weather reports

www.nws.noaa.gov

The National Oceanic and Atmospheric Administration provides detailed information on weather conditions in the United States.

www.wunderground.com

Reports on U.S. cities and states

www.weather.com

The Weather Channel's on-line service

Women travelers

www.Journeywoman.com

"An online travel resource just for women"

Travel Newsletters and Information

Whether or not you have special needs, your local public library is a rich source for newsletters relating to travel. Specialized subjects include diabetes, dialysis, special-needs travelers, adventure travel, and many more. The library's resources may be available in house or on-line; ask the reference librarian for assistance.

Travel Medicine, Inc., founded in 1989 by Stuart R. Rose, M.D., is a well-known resource for travel medicine information including travel clinics, country-specific disease information, and a plethora of travel products and medical kits. It is especially known for its line of Fight Bite insect repellents, including DEET and non-DEET repellents and permethin fabric treatment for clothes. A new, improved mosquito netting is also available. Dr. Rose's book, *International Travel Guide,* is one of the best practical books on travel medicine. For information contact:

Travel Medicine, Inc.
369 Pleasant Street
Northampton, MA 01060
(800) TRAV–MED (872–8633)
(413) 584–9254
Fax (413) 584–6656
www.travelmed.com

Shoreland has published travel information resources, including excellent newsletters, for travel medicine practitioners and clinics since 1986. Its Travax En Compass Web site has a rich library of travel health information for health professionals for an annual subscription rate. There are articles on many related travel health topics as well. Shoreland also covers some of the Travax information for the general public at www.tripprep.com. For information contact:

Shoreland
2401 North Mayfair Road, Suite 309
Milwaukee, WI 53226
(800) 433–5256
(414) 290–1900
Fax (414) 290–1907
www.shoreland.com

Travel Bookstores and Other Resources

Most book vendors, both stores and on-line services, recognize the importance of the travel market and stock an assortment of titles, but you will find the best selection and the most knowledgeable staff in stores that specialize in resources for the traveler. Check the yellow pages for specialty stores in your area or look for "travel books" on-line. For your convenience a number of independent travel bookstores are listed here.

Book Passage
51 Tamal Vista Boulevard
Corte Madera, CA 94925
(800) 999–7909
Fax (415) 924–3838
www.bookpassage.com

California Map & Travel Center
3312 Pico Boulevard
Santa Monica, CA 90405
(310) 396–6277
Fax (310) 392–8785
www.mapper.com

Distant Lands
56 South Raymond Avenue
Pasadena, CA 91105
(800) 310–3220
Fax (626) 398–7079
www.distantlands.com

Explore, Inc.
620 West Lincoln Way
Ames, IA 50010
(515) 232–8843
Fax (515) 232–4159
www.toexplore.com

Going in Style
609 Stanford Shopping Center
Palo Alto, CA 94304
(800) 637–8953
Fax (650) 356–0370
www.goinginstyle.com

Passenger Stop
812 Kenilworth Drive
Towson, MD 21204
(800) 261–5888
www.passengerstop.com

Powell's Travel Store
701 SW Sixth Avenue
Portland, OR 97204
(800) 546–5025
Fax (503) 228–7062
www.powells.com

The Savvy Traveller

310 South Michigan Avenue

Chicago, IL 60604

(888) 666–6200

Fax (312) 913–9866

www.thesavvytraveller.com

Travel Bug

328 South Guadalupe Street, Suite E

Santa Fe, NM 87501

(877) 438–2544

www.mapsofnewmexico.com

Travelden Books & Maps

461 South Kirkwood Road

St. Louis, MO 63122

(314) 909–6900

Fax (314) 909–6902

www.travelden.com

The Traveler

287 Winslow Way East

Bainbridge Island, WA 98110

(206) 842–4578

Fax (206) 780–2797

www.thetraveler.com

Traveler's Bookcase

8375 West Third Street

Los Angeles, CA 90048

(323) 655–1197

Fax (323) 655–1197

www.travelbooks.com

Traveler's Pack, Ltd.

9427 North May Avenue

Oklahoma City, OK 73120

(405) 755–2924

Fax (405) 755–0257

www.travelerspack.com

The Travel Store
56½ North Santa Cruz Avenue
Los Gatos, CA 95030
(800) 874–9397
Fax (408) 399–5177
www.travelitems.com

Wide World Books & Maps
4411A Wallingford Avenue North
Seattle, WA 98103
(888) 534–3453
Fax (206) 634–0558
www.travelbooksandmaps.com

Other Useful Numbers

Centers for Disease Control and Prevention (CDC)
(404) 639–3534 or (800) 311–3435
www.cdc.com

Hotel Doctor
(800) HOTEL–DR (468–3537)
This San Diego–based company lists 2,500 physicians available to call on people in hotel rooms in the United States or Canada.

MedicAlert
(800) 432–5378 or (800) 825–3785
Fax (209) 669–2495

State Department
The State Department's travel warnings, consular information sheets, and public announcements are available by phone. Hear recorded information at (202) 647–5225 using a Touch-Tone telephone. To receive information by automated telefax, phone (202) 647–3000 and follow the instructions.

If you need to inquire about "an actual life or death emergency, or require other assistance not addressed in the U.S. Department of State's web-based material," contact the Overseas Citizens Services (OCS) or the after-hours duty officer by phone twenty-four hours a day, seven days a week at (202) 647–5225.

Travel Record
The form on the next page will be useful if you need it while away from home.

Record of Traveler's Vital Information

Name: _____

Travel dates (attach a copy of complete itinerary):_____

_____

In case of emergency, contact: _____

_____

_____

Passport number (attach a copy of first two pages of each passport): _____

_____

Driver's license number: _____

Travelers' check numbers:_____

_____

_____

Credit card types and numbers: _____

_____

_____

Physicians' names and phone numbers: _____

_____

_____

Travel agent's name and phone number: _____

_____

Relatives (name, phone number): _____

_____

_____

Nearest neighbor (name, phone number):_____

_____

House keys left with (name, phone number):_____

_____

Animals left with (name, phone number):_____

_____

Contact at place of business (name, phone number):_____

_____

Carry this information in your security pouch; leave a copy with someone you trust.

Index

R

About the Author

Marlene Coleman developed her expertise in travel medicine early in her career in response to the challenges her patients presented both before and after their local and global travels. She is a board-certified pediatrician with an emphasis in adolescent medicine and a subspecialty in travel medicine.

Dr. Coleman is also an Associate Clinical Professor of Family Medicine at the University of Southern California Medical School and an attending physician at the California Institute of Technology, helping to keep students healthy as they study, lecture, and travel all over the world.

She serves on the Board of Trustees and Quality Review Board for the Cooperative of American Physicians–Mutual Protection Trust, a medical malpractice company. As a captain in the U.S. Naval Reserve Medical Corps, Dr. Coleman was called to active duty for Operation Desert Storm, serving in Washington, D.C., at the Navy Annex to the Pentagon.

Dr. Coleman is a popular speaker on a variety of health-related topics, most particularly healthy travel with children. She received her medical degree from the University of California at Irvine Medical School and also holds a Bachelor of Science, Master of Science, and Advanced Master's in Medical Education from the University of Southern California. Dr. Coleman lives in Los Angeles with her husband.